Rush
of
Heaven

Rush
of
Heaven

One Woman's Miraculous
Encounter with Jesus

EMA McKINLEY

with Cheryl Ricker

ZONDERVAN®

ZONDERVAN

Rush of Heaven

Copyright © 2014 by Ema L. McKinley

This title is also available as a Zondervan ebook. Visit www.zondervan.com/ebooks.

Requests for information should be addressed to:

Zondervan, 3900 *Sparks Dr. SE, Grand Rapids, Michigan 49546*

Library of Congress Cataloging-in-Publication Data

McKinley, Ema, 1946- author.
    Rush of heaven / Ema McKinley ; with Cheryl Ricker.
      pages. cm
    Includes bibliographical references and index.
    ISBN 978-0-310-33890-1 (hardcover : alk. paper)
    1. McKinley, Ema, 1946- 2. Reflex sympathetic dystrophy—Patients—Religious life.
   3. Healing—Religious aspects—Christianity. I. Ricker, Cheryl, author. II. Title.
    BV4910.337.M35 2014
    231.7'3092—dc23
    [B]   2014016659

Some names and descriptive details have been changed.

Cheryl Ricker, "In Tune," in *A Friend in the Storm* (Grand Rapids, MI: Zondervan, 2010).

"Jesus Loves the Little Children," original lyrics by C. Herbert Woolston (1856–1927), music by George F. Root (1820–1895).

Published in association with the literary agency of WordServe Literary Group, Ltd., www.wordserveliterary.com

Cover design: Faceout Studio
Cover photo: Michael Lok / Getty Images®
Interior design: Katherine Lloyd, The DESK

First Printing August 2014 / Printed in the United States of America

For the One who understands pain
beyond disfigurement

Whoever has my commands and keeps them is the one who loves me. The one who loves me will be loved by my Father, and I too will love them and show myself to them.

Contents

Prologue

December 24, 2011

The wind picked up, cutting into my skin like razor blades. I took one last look at the stars, and with my upper body hanging in its usual place, ninety degrees to the left of my wheelchair, I grabbed my wheel with my working hand and used my good foot to drag forward.

You can do it, baby.

I cranked open the oversized door, but my wheels got stuck on the threshold. Groaning, I tried again.

It's worth the extra independence, I told myself.

Every night after my caregivers went home, I unlatched my seat belt so I could move a bit and get a better grip on the wheel. Made it easier to try to pull this kind of stunt.

One last tug and my sixty-five-year-old body broke loose into the kitchen, smack into the smell of sloppy joes and ham. My caregiver had moved them from the slow cookers to the fridge before leaving, and in nineteen hours, the boys would be over to dig in after their Christmas Eve service.

I looked at my table with its place mats, plates, goblets, and candles. Everything sang Christmas. Each year I came up with a different theme and kept it hush until our big celebration. Until then, I wouldn't even let Jason, my forty-one-year-old, into the house.

I pulled my crooked body to the lighted archway in my living room so I could gaze at my Christmas tree with its gift-box ornaments and twinkling lights.

This birthday theme is for you, Jesus. You're our honored guest.

Rest. I ached to enter it completely, but whenever I tried, pain cut into my deepest sleep. Bound to a wheelchair 24-7, I could at least close my eyes and dream.

I'd told my sons, "You're going to have to work for your presents this year." Jeff, my thirty-eight-year-old, would have to sing for a friend down the street. Jason would phone a few relatives, and my grandsons would follow my clues. I smiled at my sneaky ways. This would be one Christmas we'd never forget.

I took a deep breath and started down the hall, inch by inch, pull by pull. Wheeling into my office, Savannah welcomed me with a meow.

"Cheery in here, isn't it, girl?"

My collector dolls stood on the shelves close to the ceiling. We didn't get many Christmas gifts as farm kids, but everyone always pulled together to buy me a doll. These fancy ones had come from Jeff and Jason, and oh, how they kept the memories alive.

Parking under my desk, I flicked on my computer. I might be a tough old bird, but at least I could encourage people on Facebook. Excitedly, I scrolled to my latest post. December 17, 2011:

Matthew 1:23:
" 'The virgin will conceive and give birth to a son, and they will
call him Immanuel' (which means 'God with us')."

In the midst of this wonderful Christmas season, my friends, we must all remember that God is always with us wherever we are. Blessings to you!

What a promise. Immanuel ... God with us. *Lord Jesus, may everyone who reads this post find lasting hope in you.*

What should I write next? Show me, Lord.

A verse from Matthew popped into my head: "With God all things are possible." I liked it, but where was the reference? Scanning my room sideways, I spotted my Bible on my second desk. I'd have to back up to grab it, but no big deal. I did it all the time.

Reaching for my wheel, I pushed off with my right foot while turning. But I must not have pulled back far enough, because my wheelchair caught on the side of my desk. Frustrated, I gave it another quick push—and my right wheel came off the floor ...

No—!

My heart leaped as my body flew.

Pain exploded when the curve of my neck slammed the floor, crushing it against the bend. Fire shot through my spine.

My crooked foot got pinned somewhere behind my right leg, and my left arm lay trapped beneath me. All I could see of it was my big club fist, looking lifeless and useless in front of my face.

Fear gripped me. I couldn't move. Couldn't straighten my left leg. The slightest attempt spiked pain. The phone sat on my desk, but I couldn't reach it.

"Help!" It was no use. My neighbors in the townhome beside me were away for Christmas. My heart sank. Only one person could hear my gut-wrenching cries.

Jesus!

Surely, he'd rescue me.

Savannah kept sticking her whiskery head in my face and leaving the room howling. I'd never heard such a desperate cry from a cat.

Jesus, is this how you're going to take me home?

I tried to focus on heaven, but sickness bit into me. I thought I'd experienced every level of pain, but I was wrong. So wrong.

Jesus, where are you? My helper, my Savior, my lifeline.

The words got stuck in my mouth. I could only keep screaming his name.

"Jesus!"

I imagined him taking those nails. Yielding to blow after blow. Every time I called, I knew he heard me. He had to. He'd listened to me all my life, even when nobody else did. Time after time, he'd rescued me, and he'd never stopped loving me. Even now, in my darkest hour, he wouldn't let me down.

The clock on my desk seemed to mock me. Thoughts of loved ones came and left. Who would find me? Who would call 911?

Hour sank into endless hour and the pain raged on. Trapped by my own body, I could only keep screaming his name. Over and over, I screamed it, from my raw, parched throat.

"Jesus!"

Eight and a half hours passed and I was still fully awake.

Jesus, is this what it feels like to die?

Suddenly, without warning, something began to change. Something began to shift in the atmosphere.

Out of nowhere, I heard it—loud and reverberating, roaring and growing like the wind. My heart raced.

Distant and close at the same time, it consumed my whole house, closing in on me ...

A powerful presence. Like I wasn't alone.

What in the world?

I held my breath ...

The Accident

I carried a squirt gun to work. Nothing fancy, just a little one I kept hidden in the pocket of my khaki store pants—to spice things up, really. Sometimes I aimed at coworkers on the other side of the shelves. Other times I shot from the ladder in my Health and Beauty section and ran back down to hide. If someone looked, I'd scrunch up my eyes and pretend to concentrate on my products.

Once a lady stared at the ceiling as if we'd sprung a leak. I could hardly hold my laughter.

I could use some of that same stress relief right about now. Being the Saturday before Easter, we were all a little on edge.

Lana waved as she passed. "Still need a ride?"

"Absolutely," I said. "I'll meet you by the front door at closing."

My husband, Eddie, usually picked me up, but tonight he had to fetch Jeff from college. I hadn't seen our son since Christmas, so my heart sped up just thinking about him. Knowing me, I'd be bouncing off the walls until the precise moment they walked in the door after midnight.

"Excuse me . . . ma'am?"

Turning, I faced the same petite lady I'd helped the day before. I could still picture her adorable bouncy-haired little girls twirling for me in their frilly new Easter dresses.

13

"I came back to thank you," she said, nervously. "You went out of your way to find us those dresses—so here. I brought you a gift certificate from Baker's Square. I hope you like pie."

I laughed. "You didn't need to do that. I loved helping your sweeties. But thanks. I'll definitely enjoy the pumpkin pie."

My eyes brimmed as I pocketed her gift. *Thank you, Jesus. You sure know how to put an extra skip in my step.* And me oh my—with all the last-minute Easter shoppers, I needed every extra skip I could get. Products leaped off the shelves like hot potatoes. People changed their minds a dozen times before dropping off goodies all over the place. And boy, did the questions fly: Where are the baskets? The chocolates? The roasters?

Just then Rick, my manager, whizzed by. "Jet's in the air."

Everybody knew what it meant when the manager said, "Jet's in the air." It meant the big guys from Garretts' headquarters were coming on Monday to do an inspection.

I grabbed a pencil and paper and zoomed up and down my aisles, recording all the products I needed from storage. Every shelf had to be filled; every endcap lined to perfection.

I kicked into powerhouse mode. And by the time ten o'clock rolled around, I'd already unloaded my boxes of liquid products from the trolley and heaped them in the middle of my section floor. I hated leaving them like that, but I'd be right back. I just had to grab my paper products from the second storage room. Then I could put everything away at once.

Warmth greeted me the instant I pushed back those double doors. It came from the old drum heater above the loft where I needed to get my products. As I stepped up the ladder, heat gripped me. And when I finally reached the loft, I groaned. Someone had stacked the boxes almost to the ceiling! What was the deal? Had we received an extra big shipment and the stock guy didn't know what to do with them? Either way, I knew what I had to do. I had to climb over those boxes to get my products.

As I worked my way up the first layer, I rewrote my job description: *Must be able to act like a monkey*—because that's what we felt like whenever we did this. Boxes shifted and shook beneath my weight.

Keep going, I told myself. It won't be long before you're home waiting for Jeff. And soon you'll be catching up on all the thrills of college life.

If only my other son, Jason, could be with us too, but he was in South Carolina working on F-16 fighters in the Air Force. At least he'd soon be home for his wedding.

I wiped my brow. After climbing three levels of boxes, I still couldn't find the right bar codes to match the items on my list. Where were they? Where was that crazy Kleenex?

I thought about working my way back down—maybe hunting for a stock guy—but with everybody so busy, it hardly made sense. Besides, I was already halfway up. Sometimes you just need to get the job done and over with.

Crawling up the next two layers of boxes, the air grew hotter. "Who needs this?" I grumbled.

Finally reaching the top, I stole a breath. The Kleenex had to be there. I'd grab what I needed, hurry back down, put it all away, and catch my ride with Lana.

But where was the right bar code?

I held out my arms for balance and headed for the boxes by the wall. Don't look down, I told myself. I had to be at least twenty-five feet from the floor. Wobbling, I grabbed one of the steel vertical beams for support. Thick boards jutted out, leaving a thin open space between the wall and me.

That's when I saw it. The big round drum heater in the ceiling! I'd never seen it so close. It couldn't have been more than four feet away.

Before I even had time to think, it fired up with a roar. I was staring into the bright blaze of the flame. Heat blasted my body.

And everything went black.

Pain

April 12, 1993

I opened my eyes to a dim-lit room and wanted only to close them. My head felt like someone had whacked it with a crowbar. My foot and leg—like they'd been battered, ripped apart, and pressed back together again. Wires snaked out of my hospital gown, connecting me to a heart monitor. An IV stuck out of my bruised, swollen hand.

From the corner of my eye, I saw someone beside me.

Jeff. My heart sank. "Honey ..."

He jumped to his feet. "Mom ... you're awake!"

I dragged a hand over my forehead and felt a huge goose egg of a bump. "What in the world?"

He shook his head. "Hold still. I need to grab a doctor. I said I'd let them know as soon as you woke up. We've all been so worried."

He backed out of the room, and I slowly peeked under the sheets. No way. My foot had become swollen, discolored, and crooked. Bright stripes lined my leg as if someone had taken their fingernails and clawed me from my knee to the middle of my thigh. The pain told me something much worse had happened.

I blinked into focus the doctor who suddenly appeared beside me.

"Hi, Ema. I'm Dr. Howard White."

"Hi." I sounded gravelly, but it didn't keep him from smiling.

"It's good to see you. You've been unconscious a long time."

"I have? For how long?"

A nurse straightened my bed sheets. "It's Monday. You've been out since Saturday night."

My mind reeled. Easter had come and gone and I'd missed it? How sad. Life had gone on while I was lost in some kind of never-never land.

"You sound so far away," I told her. "I can hardly hear you."

The nurse nodded. "That's common for a concussion, but don't worry. We'll take good care of you. You should be back to normal in no time."

The doctor grinned like he had a secret. "Ema, I've been keeping a close eye on you. Even when you didn't know it."

His voice sounded soothing. Almost familiar. His words struck me like something Jesus would say: *Ema, I've always been close.*

He shone a flashlight in my eyes and checked my pupils. "Do you remember what happened?"

Just then, pain gripped me and I grimaced.

"It's okay," the nurse said, patting my arm. "There's no rush. We can wait."

My eyes went to the ceiling as I tried to reach for thoughts. "I was at work. There was a loft ... Oh, I don't know. I can't remember." I sucked in a breath and brought my hand to my head.

"Don't worry," the nurse said. "You can tell us the rest later. We've connected you to a morphine pump, so feel free to push the button whenever you need more relief. It should give you a few good pushes an hour."

I normally hated medicine, but all I could think was, *When can I next push the button?*

Over the next several hours, doctors came and went, putting me through a slew of tests. I breathed a sigh of relief when they finally left the room. At last, Jeff and I could be alone. I held his hands as we shared a smattering of prayers and quiet thoughts. More than anything, I ached to wipe the pain from his eyes.

"I'm so sorry." My words sounded helpless. Pathetic. Like some-one had stolen the sails out of my voice and still left the weight of an ocean. We'd looked forward to this spring break for ages, and now this? How would I ever make it up to him?

He kissed my cheek. "I love you, Mom." He held me in his eyes until mine clouded over. "Where does it hurt most?"

"Let's see. My head and hand are screaming, but I also have a split-ting foot and leg ache."

He'd heard my stories over the years, so he knew I had a high tolerance for pain. When I was pregnant with his older brother, Jason, I labored in the hospital for three days straight, refusing all pain medi-cine. And who could blame me? In my first trimester, my nearly retired doctor had prescribed certain pills to stop my bleeding. When they didn't work, he told me I could lose the baby. Horrified, I hightailed it to a different doctor for a second opinion. When I showed him the pills, he turned beet red. "You don't want to be taking these." And with that, he flung the bottle into the trash.

"What's wrong with the pills?" I said, heart pounding. "They won't hurt the baby, will they?"

He cleared his throat. "Well, they're similar to another drug that causes birth defects."

My knees went weak as I cried out to God. *Please, may this baby be normal.* I prayed that same prayer every day until my due date. Even more after the date came and left. It passed me by three and a half weeks! A cruel joke, I thought. The big day did finally come, however. And the first thing I did when I saw my sweet little Jason was count his fingers and toes and whisper a heartfelt, *Thank you, Jesus!*

Just like I whispered now as I pushed the morphine button with one hand and squeezed Jeff's hand with the other: *Thank you, Jesus, for my amazing sons.*

Jeff's lips curved into a smile, and I let myself sink back into my pillow. Where had all the years gone? I remembered being his age, nine-teen, out of high school, eager to take on the world and get married.

A chill swept the room. Eddie. Where was he? Surely he hadn't left Jeff all alone to deal with this by himself. The poor guy didn't even know when or if I'd wake up.

"Honey, has your dad been here?"

He stiffened. "Yeah, he stopped by at the beginning, but he had to go. You know Dad. He gets tired."

Clenching my teeth, I didn't know what to say. I was too tired to pursue it anyway. The pain kept pressing in. It pressed with such fury that I was in and out of it. Bless my son's heart, he stayed at my side the whole time.

The next day, a nurse poked into the room. "Up for visitors? They're from Garretts."

I ran my fingers through my hair. "Sure. Send 'em in." I rubbed Jeff's hand. "Honey, why don't you go get some rest?"

He hugged me and traded places with Rita and Peter.

"What a relief to see you're okay," Rita said. She wasn't her normal bubbly self. She sounded more strained. "Here. I brought you an Easter basket with a few goodies."

"Thanks," I said. "Happy Easter." I had to inwardly laugh at the irony. What was so happy about it? For a few minutes, I made small talk with my friends. Then it struck me: "You guys were there. You can tell me what happened."

They exchanged looks and at last Peter drew in a breath. "Kyle found you. We were all ready to go home. Then, in the last second, Kyle saw a stray clothes rack and decided to push it into the storage room. That's when he found you."

I held his gaze. "What did he see?"

His jaw stiffened as he hesitated. "He saw your hand — dangling down from the loft."

"Sheesh," I said, shivering. "Sounds like a scene from a horror movie. What else did he see? I mean, what happened next?"

He swallowed. "Kyle ran up the ladder. You sure you're ready for this?"

"Ready and waiting."

"Okay ... Kyle found you hanging upside down by your foot and leg."

The air grew tight. "Go on," I said, refusing to back down. I wanted to hear all of it. I had to.

"Your leg had gotten completely twisted around. Your foot had gotten jammed between boxes and boards. It must have been like that the whole time."

What did he mean by *the whole time*? Something didn't sound quite right. I looked at Rita. "When did Kyle find me? I mean ... what time was it?"

She sucked in a breath. "After midnight. Around 12:45."

My mind reeled ... 12:45? I'd climbed into the loft just shortly after ten. That could only mean one thing: While everybody else was getting ready for the inspection, I was hanging upside down—for two and a half hours.

My mouth went dry. "So everybody was still there the whole time?"

Peter shifted. "Nobody could find you. We thought you'd left. That's what everybody said. That you'd gone home early."

Gone home early? The words hit like a punch. We were a team. We helped each other during closing, and we had an end-of-the-day rule that nobody left until *everybody* was ready to leave. Matter of fact, we followed that rule to a tee. How could they possibly presume I'd leave without clocking out? I always clocked out. And what about Lana? I never canceled my ride. And my floor? Goodness, everyone knew I was a perfectionist. How could they think I'd leave everything undone, in such a mess? It didn't make sense. Right now, however, I hurt too much to dwell on it. I was just too drained.

"Thanks again for the Easter basket," I said. "I think I'd better rest now."

The pain continued to grow worse, so I asked a nurse if the morphine pump was working.

"Looks good to me," she said.

Doctors and nurses filed in and out, examining me, doing tests, and asking questions. "My head feels like it's in a big drum," I told them.

"I'm sure it does," the nurse said, sympathetically. "It's a wonder you're even alive."

❉

On Wednesday, Shanda, my personnel manager, walked in with two of the bigwigs from corporate headquarters. "How do you feel?" she asked.

I thought for a second. "Like a broken piece of glass."

We rattled on for a while about my condition, but their sympathy soon dissolved into questions. I shuddered when I figured out the granddaddy question behind them all: How in the world could something so terrible happen in *their* store?

As I told them about the boxes almost touching the ceiling and the heater blasting my body with heat, they looked a little heat blasted themselves. Something told me there'd be a lot more to this discussion.

❉

My tests and X-rays came back normal. No fractures, breaks, or red flags. Confusion lined everybody's faces. If everything faired so fine and dandy, why in the world was my foot so twisted with pain?

Eight days passed and they sent in a therapist, a middle-aged woman, to work on me. "I'm going to try to desensitize your foot by rubbing it with a terry cloth towel."

If I'd known what that would do, I wouldn't have given in to it so easily. The instant she moved the terry cloth towel across my foot, I let out a piercing scream. Two nurses stepped in to see what was wrong.

"She's fine," the therapist said.

Oh, no she's not! I wanted to shout—but I hurt too much to speak. What in the world was wrong with me?

When they put my foot and leg in a cast, I mistakenly thought they might actually leave me alone for a while, but no, not at all. Instead, they sent me to the physical therapy room to see Vance Wade.

"Let's get you moving on these crutches," he said, crossing his arms in front of his tall, lean body.

As I held myself up, my eyes pleaded with him. "My foot's throbbing. Do you mind if we take it slow?"

He swatted the air and grabbed a second pair of crutches to give me the big demo. Goodness, the way he kicked off on those things, you'd think he was trying to win a three-legged race at a church picnic.

"Your turn," he said.

I took a few cautious steps and glanced at him.

"Keep going," he said.

Tears rolled down my face.

"Don't be afraid," he said. "The crutches will hold you up." I took a few more steps and he did a hand clap. "Okay, it's now time for our special staircase."

I stared at the six practice steps in the corner. "Really? Don't you think I should get a little more used to the floor?"

He cleared his throat. "Look, the sooner you do this, the sooner we'll be finished."

I wanted to scream, but even more I wanted to be done with it. So, gritting my teeth, I anchored my crutches and took that first step up the stairs.

Lord, give me strength.

He most certainly did, and this became my ongoing prayer over the next few days until they released me.

I should have been celebrating the big day. After all, I'd just spent two crazy weeks in the hospital. But my foot hurt more than ever, so I hobbled out the door feeling misunderstood and confused—oblivious to the monster growing beneath the surface.

Diagnosis

"Why don't they hurry up?" Eddie said it behind his newspaper as we slumped in our umpteenth waiting room.

"Ema Lano?"

Grabbing my crutches, we followed a receptionist down a hall to a large room that curtained off into several smaller rooms. There, a young therapist extended his hand. "I'm Wayne Jerome. Have you ever heard of TENS? A transcutaneous electrical nerve stimulator?"

I shook my head. "A who?"

Eddie watched with fascination as Wayne stuck patches around my crooked foot and ankle where the cast used to be. "This will stimulate the affected area by sending brain signals to block off the pain."

"Sounds delightful," I said.

Wayne kept his hand near the dial, making adjustments. "Feel that?"

I laughed. "I didn't even know you'd turned it on."

He wrinkled his brow and made more adjustments. "You'll feel it now because I turned it up. Let me know if it's too much."

I waited, but didn't feel the slightest vibration, only his eyes on my foot and his voice in my ears. "Well?"

"Well, I still don't feel anything."

He bit on his lip and reached for the machine. "Unbelievable. We'll increase the intensity then. Ready? Here it goes. Feel anything?"

"No, not a thing."

His eyes widened. "Okay then, we'll crank it all the way to the top."

I kept my eyes on his fidgeting fingers as he pushed the button. "Still nothing," I said. "Not even a tingle."

He laughed nervously, then turned to Eddie. "Mind if I borrow your arm? I don't think this machine is working, so I'd like to test it on you."

My husband shrugged. "Sure."

Wayne arranged the patches the same way he'd done on me. "We'll start with the lowest setting, okay? Ready? Here goes."

"Ah!" Eddie screamed, bolting out of his chair. He shot out so fast you would have thought his rear was on fire.

"Wow," Wayne said, shaking his head. "I thought for sure the machine was broken."

I struggled to stay calm. Everything in me wanted to bolt away too. If the machine wasn't broken, then where did that leave me? Was I the broken one? I sure felt like it. Goodness, I'd never felt like such a stranger to myself—to my own body. My nerves and muscles weren't communicating with my brain. I didn't get it. Why would a terry cloth towel make me scream bloody murder and a nerve stimulator do absolutely nothing?

＊

Over the next week or so, my foot turned a lovely shade of fire-engine red with a bright purple blotch in the middle. In just a few minutes, it could go from freezing like ice to as hot as an electric blanket. My original swollenness had morphed into full-blown edema stretching all the way up my calf.

Dr. Paul Clause, my primary-care doctor, needed more information to diagnose my condition. So he sent me to Dr. Stephen Noll, a specialist in lower extremities, for more testing.

The thirty-something-year-old doctor wore a thin smile and kind eyes. "This may feel a little uncomfortable," Dr. Noll said, "but we're going to put your leg in this big blue boot and pump it up to drain some of the fluid."

He pumped me up so tight that he nearly squeezed the yahoo out of me! When I caught my breath, I had a question. "My son's getting married in about eight weeks. Do you have any idea if I'll be better by then?"

He blew out a gust of air. "Hard to say. I'm working on your case with your primary-care physician and a couple others. I think we'll need to send you for more testing before we can confirm anything."

More testing? I was beginning to hate the word. Okay, so what was that verse I'd learned way back in Sunday school? "Consider it pure joy, my brothers and sisters, whenever you face trials of many kinds, because you know that the testing of your faith produces perseverance" (James 1:2–3).

Hey, God, whatever you're trying to produce in me, can you kindly produce it a little faster? I'd really like to get this testing behind me.

After a bone scan and a couple other tests, I sat in Dr. Noll's office, wondering exactly what hoop they'd have me jump through next.

"How are you doing?" Dr. Noll asked.

"As good as can be expected. It's hard to believe it's been forty days since the accident." I pointed upward. "It's a good thing God's holding me up."

He smiled. "I'm glad you've got your faith. Well ... I think we finally know what we're dealing with here."

"Phew." I sighed loudly. "Now that's an answer to prayer."

"Oh, I wouldn't get too excited about it yet." He moved closer and tapped on his clipboard. "From what we've put together, it looks like you have reflex sympathetic dystrophy."

"Muscular dystrophy?" The words hung between us in the air. I'd worked with several people who had MD, and I knew just how horrible it could be.

He shook his head. "No, not muscular dystrophy. You have reflex sympathetic dystrophy, or RSD. It's also known as complex regional pain syndrome, or CRPS. It's an unusual and painful disorder of the sympathetic nervous system, and it affects people to different degrees. It attacks the nerves, skin, muscles, blood vessels, and bones — sometimes all at once. Oh, and it's often caused by trauma, which makes sense in your case."

"Is it ... curable?"

"Sometimes, with the right physical therapy. And that's our next plan. Therapy and medication for the pain."

"Um, my son's getting married on July tenth."

"Don't worry," he said. "We'll stick with outpatient therapy for now. We won't start you on inpatient therapy until after the wedding."

Good. God, in his mercy, would probably heal me before then. I earnestly prayed he would. "Is there anything else I need to know about RSD?" I asked the doctor. "Please. You can be frank with me."

"Well, you might not like this, Ema. But RSD is right up there in the McGill Pain Index. It's at the top of the chart. So I guarantee you that you'll need some good strong steady support in the days ahead."

My mind reeled like a windmill. Could God possibly be using all this to bring Eddie and me closer together? Now *that* would be a miracle.

I Do

July 10, 1993

The organ played "He Leadeth Me" while bridesmaids and grooms-men walked their separate aisles, joining each other at the front. When the music changed, everyone rose to their feet and turned to the back.

Light streamed through the window, catching her face. I held my breath as Tara, my soon-to-be daughter-in-law, stepped out in her long, flowing white gown.

Pain took a backseat as my finger went snap-happy on my camera. I always loved taking wedding pictures — something I'd even been hired to do a few times — but this was tops. Nothing melted my heart like seeing my son take Tara's hands and make promises before God and the relatives. What mother didn't dream of this moment? And if God saw fit, somewhere in the future there'd be grandchildren.

Daddy gave me a wink. He looked sharp and stately in his charcoal suit. The cousins, aunts, and uncles beamed and dabbed their eyes. We were a close family. Two of Mom's sisters had married three of Daddy's brothers, giving me double cousins on both sides. Double blessings.

Whenever we got together like this, we reminisced about family reunions at Grandma and Grandpa Reeves' farm. We remembered their Bible stories and hand-clapping sing-alongs. The kids took turns bouncing on Grandpa's knees while Aunt Jean pounded the piano, and everybody belted out hymns like the ones the organist played today.

Jason's eyes twinkled as they locked on Tara's. What a beauty with her shoulder-length raven hair beneath her veil.

When the pastor said, "For better, for worse," I glanced at Eddie, who looked as serious as always. I wondered if he was still upset about what happened before the ceremony. While we were taking family pictures, he stepped away to grab a Coke from the church fridge. Knowing we were on a tight schedule, the pastor yelled at him. "Eddie, get with the program!" Of course, I'd blushed for him, but that was Eddie. Always plodding around, doing his own thing.

He was that way with the boys too. Often ignoring them. Once when they were little, they reached for him with stars in their eyes and homemade Christmas gifts in their hands. "Here, Daddy. We made this for you. Do you like it?" Absently, he took their gifts, barely gave them a glance, and dropped them to the floor. Then, as if nothing happened, he walked off into his own world, never even bothering to pick them up.

Even the memory crushed me—seeing the boys' eyes cloud over. Helpless, I ran to the bathroom, crying out to God. *I can't take it anymore. He's neglecting the children.* That's when the Comforter came. In that sliver of a moment, he slipped into my thinking, with love, truth, and understanding: *Ema, what you feel is the same way my heart breaks for all my children when they're hurting. I hurt when they hurt. Just like I rejoice when they rejoice.*

How refreshing to know that God rejoiced with me now. Because as Jason and Tara exchanged rings, I felt waves of their happiness. So God must have felt them too.

The pastor gave Jason a nod. "You may now kiss the bride." The church broke into cheers while my happy finger kept clicking.

As soon as Jason and Tara moved to the receiving line, I hobbled behind them. And then I followed them outside by the trees and flowers. Such a picture-perfect day.

I got so caught up in capturing their love and laughter that I set down my crutches. Jason gave me a sideways look. "Mom. Should you be doing that?"

"Oh, I'll be fine."

I wouldn't let anything spoil this day. Not my pain. Not Eddie being bawled out. Not even my upcoming inpatient therapy.

Aggressive

Dr. Derek Reeve wore a white coat over a business suit and sat on his desk, instructing his therapist. "Dig in, Darlene. Work that foot and make it straight."

Darlene sat on a tiny-legged stool, gripping my foot in her lap. Giving it gusto, she pushed my heel one way and my toes the other.

"Please!" I said. "Can you just let me catch my breath?" In my wildest dreams, I never imagined inpatient therapy would be like this.

"I know it hurts," Dr. Reeve said, "but you've got to do it."

His words jarred, but not as much as the pain. Darlene breathed heavily, squeezing up and down my big swollen calf. The therapy took so much out of her that she needed to rest her hands.

Dr. Reeve shot her a look that sent her back to work. And just when I thought things couldn't get worse, a second therapist strolled in.

"Fabulous," Dr. Reeve said. "Crystal, you take the foot. Darlene, you get the leg."

Crystal's fingers attacked my crooked foot—twisting and flattening it like a helpless piece of dough. Tears streamed down my face as I cupped my trembling hand over my mouth, trying to suppress my cries.

"I'm sorry," Darlene said. I could tell she hated this, and I loved her for it. Yes, they did all this to help people, but how on earth could they do it day after day? Did they even have a clue about my pain? If RSD was so unusual and unique, wasn't it possible they didn't understand what they were dealing with?

Dr. Reeve hopped to his feet and gave me a smile. "That's it for the day." The two therapists instantly backed off to stretch their muscles. Me? I grabbed my crutches, hobbled back to my room, and threw up.

Jesus, where are you? What did I do to deserve this?

I resented my thoughts and where they were heading, but I felt too weak to snap out of them on my own, so I sought comfort in Scripture, in Philippians 4:13: "I can do all this through him who gives me strength."

You need to fight back, I told myself. You need to stay above the water. Grabbing my Bible, I turned to Ephesians 6:10–13:

> Finally, be strong in the Lord and in his mighty power. Put on the full armor of God, so that you can take your stand against the devil's schemes. For our struggle is not against flesh and blood, but against the rulers, against the authorities, against the powers of this dark world and against the spiritual forces of evil in the heavenly realms. Therefore put on the full armor of God, so that when the day of evil comes, you may be able to stand your ground, and after you have done everything, to stand.

I'd probably read that passage a few hundred times in my life, but in my weakness, it quenched me like a drink on a hot day, giving me strength. Sure, Satan aimed at me with lies and discouragement, but I didn't have to let him scrunch my armor!

Jesus, I don't know where you're taking me through this tunnel, but no matter what happens, please help me stand brave and tall—at least on the inside.

Burn

August 2, 1993

As Daddy stood over my bed with a big farmer hand on mine, he asked God to be with me. *"Thank you for your love and protection that never leaves us, Father. And thank you for working good into everything because Ema has been called by your purpose. No matter what happens, we give you the praise. In Jesus' name."*

Daddy kept his eyes on my ballooned-up leg. "I can't see them doing therapy with your leg looking like this."

Minutes later, a nurse walked in, stretching and pulling on a long white sock. "This is a compression sock," she said. "Dr. Reeve ordered it to help reduce your edema so we can get you back in therapy."

Daddy and I exchanged looks.

"Are you ready?" she said. "We're going to work this on you."

I shrugged. "Go ahead."

As the sock rolled over my toes, I dug my fingers into the sides of the bed.

"Hang in there," she said. Higher and higher she hiked it, up and around my big swollen leg, practically suffocating it.

"Very good," she said, backing out of the room. "Call me if you need anything, okay?"

I can handle this, I told myself, trying to breathe. Two minutes later, however, the sock bore into me like a branding iron.

"It's burning!" I screamed.

32

The nurse ran back in. "What on earth?"

"Take it off," I ordered. "Hurry—it's burning!"

"Did you just say it's *burning*?" she said, hand on hip. "Now that doesn't make sense."

"Please," I begged. "Take it off. If you don't, I will. It's burning my skin clear through!"

"Really . . . ," she said slowly. "Well, the doctor ordered this treatment, so if you're tempted to take it off, I should probably stay here and make sure that you don't."

Daddy crossed his arms. "Ema's in pain. Please take off the sock or at least let me do it."

The nurse puffed out her chest and gave me an exasperated look. "Listen, I know it *feels* like it's burning, but it's just a compression sock. It'll make you better."

Who was she trying to kid? It hurt so much I couldn't help myself. I broke into sobs.

Daddy's face turned as red as a crab apple. "Look . . . are you going to keep ignoring her or are you going to do something?"

The nurse threw up her hands. "All right, I'll check with the doctor."

A minute later, she stepped back in. "All is well. Dr. Reeve says we can take it off and check it out."

I bit into my lip as she peeled it back. Then the breath got sucked out of me. In several places, my leg was burned raw! Her fingers trembled as she dragged down the rest of it.

"Aahh . . ." I groaned. "It's taking my skin off!"

"I am *so* sorry." Her voice cracked as she shook her head. "Must be an allergic reaction. Um, there's really no other explanation." She pulled out some kind of wire contraption and tented it over my leg. "This will keep the sheets from touching the burn."

Disappointment fell on me like a cloud. Why couldn't people listen to me the first time?

⁎

When Dr. Reeve returned an hour later, he slid his glasses to the end of his nose and flung off my sheets. "Let's take a look," he said. A slight *hmm* escaped his throat before he spoke. "That's quite the rash."

Heat rose to my cheeks. *How dare he stare at my missing flesh and call it a rash!*

He left the room before I had a chance to protest or say anything. He left me alone with my thoughts.

Jesus, did you hear what that doctor just said to me? He doesn't know his rashes from his burns!

The next time the nurse walked in, she wore a secretive look. "I probably shouldn't tell you this," she said, "but you really stumped Dr. Reeve today. He draped himself over the nurses' desk and talked all about your burn."

"Oh, really?" I said, hungry for details. "What did he say?"

"He said, 'In my entire career, I have never seen anything remotely like it.'"

Anger squeezed in my chest.

The nurse's forehead wrinkled. "Are you okay?"

"I will be. In time."

"Well, I'm here if you need me." She tapped on my chart with her pen. "Looks like tomorrow they're giving you an epidural."

Numb

August 3, 1993

The doctor stopped what he was doing to give me his full attention. "Ema, we're going to block all the nerves in your left leg so you won't feel a thing during therapy."

"Go for it," I said with gusto.

He chuckled. "You're the kind of patient we like."

I held my breath as the needle dug into my spine. Funny how I'd survived having babies without one of these, but now I needed one to make it through physical therapy.

A minute passed. "Feel anything?"

An easy smile turned up my lips. "Both legs are numb all the way down to my toes."

"Good," he said. "That's what we want."

Two or three minutes passed before something began to stir and tingle in my left leg and crooked foot. I sucked in a breath as the stirring quickly turned into hard-core pain.

His brows knitted together. "What is it?"

"My legs. I don't feel anything in my right one. But my left one— it feels absolutely *everything*." My mind went to Wayne, the therapist with the nerve stimulator.

Oh, Lord, please may this be different than that.

The doctor checked and rechecked everything and scratched his head. "I'll tell ya what. How 'bout we give it a few hours, then see what happens?"

"Okay," I said, weakly. As if I had a choice.

Time crawled like a baby as I waited—but nothing happened.

You're still with me, aren't you, Jesus? I thought of his words in Matthew 28:20: "Surely I am with you always, to the very end of the age."

Three hours passed and the doctor looked at me expectantly. "How does it feel?"

Helpless, I shook my head. "The pain's off the charts."

He ran a hand through his hair and started for the door. "I'll be right back."

I wanted to shout, Hey, wait! Don't go! But instead I talked to the Lord: *What now? Please tell me this is just a fluke.*

Just then, someone new walked in. "Hi, I'm Dr. Wayne Barkly. I'm sorry, but I think we need to start over fresh."

My eyes widened. "Why? I mean ... did the other doctor make a mistake?"

He shook his head. "Not really a mistake. We just need to try again."

I leaned forward as he removed the old catheter. He showed confidence, that's for sure—but hadn't the other guy? My confidence, on the other hand, had seen better days. It must have drip-dropped away like the medicine hanging over my head in that little plastic bag.

The doctor double-checked his equipment. "Okay, here goes." He stuck me again, launching me right back in the waiting game.

One minute stretched into two, then three ... Relax, I told myself. Enjoy the pain melting away. And I did enjoy it—for four minutes. Then the pain hit me like a wrecking ball.

"Umm, doctor? My right leg is asleep, but my left leg is screaming bloody murder."

He shook his head in disbelief. "Can you move it for me?"

He didn't believe me! Fine, I'd show him. I wiggled my toes, daring him to double-doubt me. Clenching my teeth, I lifted and bent my puffy left leg. Woo-hoo ... Look what I can do!

He pinched the bridge of his nose. "I'll be right back."

Great, I thought. Not another one. If I chased them all away, who'd be left? I wanted to go fetch him—but my right leg was still dead to the world. I also wanted to scream, "Hey, does anybody here know about RSD? Someone? Anyone who can help me?"

I already had an idea what I'd say to the next doctor: "Hey, are you here for the leg show too?"

I ate my words, however, when Dr. Reeve strode in.

His eyes narrowed as they zoomed in on my leg, almost like he was challenging it. Slowly, weakly, I lifted it up and down, feeling about as strong as a piece of dirt. The room felt weighty and stiff like my leg.

Dr. Reeve cleared his throat. "You've been scheduled for a six-day epidural. We'd like to keep you on that schedule. Who knows—with any luck, the anesthetics might kick in before then."

I almost choked. "So that's it?"

"I'm sorry this is so difficult," he said.

Difficult? I'd seen characters in movies escape from hospitals for smaller deals.

God, I need you to remind me of your love. I need to feel your strong arms . . .

I flipped through the highlighted verses in my Bible and stopped at Deuteronomy 31:8: "The LORD himself goes before you and will be with you; he will never leave you nor forsake you. Do not be afraid; do not be discouraged."

God's arms came in the form of friends and family who drove a good distance to see me. Of course, I always had Daddy and Ellie. Ellie Miller had been a dear friend since I took a factory job fresh out of high school. God also brought me Uncle Alan, Aunt Pearl, several cousins, my brother Sam, his wife Carol, and my nephew Andrew.

Aunt Pearl couldn't stop crying. "I can't believe your epidural's not working. Oh, Ema, I hate to see you like this."

"Boy, I must look pretty bad," I said. "Should I look in a mirror?" It felt good to laugh. Faith and laughter, two of God's greatest gifts for the hurting. I just wished the potato-sized knot in my stomach would rot itself out. Worry crept into my thoughts. If RSD could do this much damage to my nerves and muscles, what could it do to the rest of me?

After everybody left, I welcomed some quiet time. No fear, I told myself. If you want to move forward, you need to face your giants. That had been my motto since I learned to swim at the age of thirty-five. Once I figured it out, I wanted to teach others. So when God gave me an opportunity, I worked at the Rec Center with handicapped kids.

They gave me fifteen-year-old Amanda, who had hydrocephalus, otherwise known as water on the brain. "One little splash and she'll freak," they warned. Seeing fear in her puppy-dog eyes only made me all the more determined to help her succeed.

We started off slow. I wheeled her chair down the ramp and gave her a chance to get used to the water. "Let's get your feet wet," I told her. After fifteen minutes, she let me hold her in the shallow end. "Good job, Amanda. You're brave."

Bit by bit, this sweet little gal with extra high eyebrows who refused to trust anybody else—trusted me. And before I knew it, I had her standing waist deep, laughing and splashing my face. The other workers couldn't get over it. Then one day, I got hit with a strange thought: "There's more to be done with Amanda."

Was that you, Lord? Because if it was, you're going to have to tell me extra loud and clear so I know exactly what you mean.

A couple weeks later, God gave me a creative idea to share with her. "Sweetie, I want you to stand on my feet." When she didn't protest, I knew we could do this. I placed my hands on her shoulders and scooted my feet under hers. Lo and behold, with Amanda's feet on mine, we walked step-by-step all over that pool.

The workers kept peeking in our direction. No one had ever tried to do anything like this with Amanda. One false move and she could go under. The more I worked with her, the more I couldn't let go of that thought: *There's more to be done with Amanda.*

One day, after Amanda walked on my feet, I asked if she'd like to float on her back. Happy squeals told me she did. Fully trusting me, she leaned all the way back until she floated like bread. That's all it took to move us to the next step.

"Amanda, do you want to stick your head under?" She laughed with excitement. Seconds later, she wasn't the only one holding her breath—but she did it! Fear didn't get the last laugh. Amanda did!

Then one day it happened. As Amanda walked on my feet, I heard a voice as clear as the water itself. This time, I *knew* who it was. It was the Holy Spirit ...

Amanda is going to walk out of this pool.

I stopped cold in my tracks. "Hold on, Amanda." I paused because I needed to think. Had I heard him correctly? Amanda couldn't walk. It wasn't possible.

She squirmed at my stillness, ready to keep moving. "Here we go," I said, trying to keep calm. Trying to ignore that voice in my head. But the more I moved with Amanda, the more I argued with myself. "No way, Amanda can't walk. It's not possible." Finally, it struck me: Wait a minute. I'm not arguing with myself. I'm arguing with God. I can't do that. If God says, *Amanda's going to walk out of this pool*, then Amanda's going to walk out of this pool!

It hit me that I had to make a choice—but would I be strong enough?

Someone blew the whistle. End of class. Great, I thought. This is it. Amanda's going to walk out of this pool.

Her caregivers sprang to action, getting her wheelchair ready to wheel down to us. I didn't have time to worry about what they'd think—but I already knew what I had to do. Carefully, I sidestepped around, turning my back to the ramp so Amanda could face forward. I wanted her to see where she'd be *walking*. It's now or never, I thought. Holding her arms, I pulled out my feet from under her.

"I've got your hands. Today, Amanda, is the day you're going to walk."

A squeal escaped her throat and one of the caregivers turned. "What are you doing?"

I didn't answer. I had to stay focused on Amanda. Then, right before my eyes, Amanda took her first step up the ramp.

Lord, help us.

One short step followed another and another until Amanda made it all the way to the top of the ramp! Her squeals of delight made me feel like I was floating.

"Amanda, what are you doing?" shouted her caregiver. Before I could do anything, the woman grabbed Amanda and plopped her into her wheelchair. Then she glared at me as if I'd lost my mind. "You shouldn't have done that. Amanda does *not* walk!"

Her words stung like needles. How could she say that when Amanda had just walked? She'd seen it herself.

Shake it off, I told myself. You obeyed God's voice—and Amanda walked!

That day proved to be a turning point in Amanda's life—and mine too. News about Amanda began to spread like wildfire. And two weeks later, I saw her using a walker!

"I can't thank you enough," her mother said, clutching her chest. "Now that you've shown us what Amanda can do, we don't see any reason to keep her confined in a wheelchair."

I thanked God for letting me be a part of Amanda's progress. I might have looked like a fruitcake in the process, but it was worth it.

Amanda's therapists started showing up at the pool to watch me work with her and take notes. The same caregiver who glared at me now waved, all friendly-like. It reminded me how people could change in a heartbeat. Good thing God never changes.

I thought about this as I lay in limbo-land waiting for the epidural to kick in so the therapists could do their therapy. It always helped to remember God's faithfulness in the past. The same God who helped me face my fears in the pool could help me face them now—even if it felt like I was in way over my head.

Partial Healing

August 9, 1993

The night hung over me like a thick, stiff blanket. After six solid days of being connected to an epidural, it never worked. This blew them away, of course, and me right along with them.

Now they had me tethered to a morphine pump, which didn't do much good either. Thank the Lord, I only had one more day left of this. Then I'd be able to kiss inpatient therapy good-bye forever.

The television flickered blue against the shadows as I meditated on Scripture, my tasty bread and butter. I loved diving into the secret place described in Isaiah 45:3: "I will give you hidden treasures, riches stored in secret places, so that you may know that I am the LORD, the God of Israel, who summons you by name." More than ever, his secret place had become my sweet place, a sacred territory where I could treasure him and learn to hear his voice more clearly.

Daddy, I need to camp under your shadow. I want a childlike faith that never doubts the strength of your arms.

Just then, the phone rattled my thoughts.

"Ema? It's Mary Lois. Did I wake you?"

My heart swelled to hear my sister's concerned voice. I laughed. "I've hardly slept since I've been here — even with sleeping pills!"

"I heard the epidural never worked," she said. "I'm sorry. But just think, soon you'll be out of there and back on your feet."

"I hope so," I said. "I just have to trust that God's watching over me."

"Oh, he is. He's always protected us, even when we were little. Remember the big woodshed?"

Goodness, how could I forget? The five of us kids played house in there. One day my older brother, Johnny, got an idea to tie a rope around the leg of a small table and stretch it clear over to the leg of the woodstove. His purpose? So we could divide the shed into rooms and have ourselves a little pretend kitchen.

While Mom's canning goods cooked in the pressure cooker, we made imaginary mud pies and cooked up a delectable story. We rushed between rooms, tickled by an imagination-land rich with crying babies, doting grandmas, and hungry visitors.

Everything was fine and dandy until Mary Lois wanted to move into Johnny's room. Without thinking, Johnny yanked the rope, toppling the stove. The next thing I knew, Mary Lois and I were flat on the floor in a sea of boiling hot water.

"Fire!" screamed Johnny, as burning logs rolled across the floor.

Mom heard our cries and burst inside. I still don't know how she got us to the kitchen. While Mom waited for the fire truck, police, and ambulance, she did the first thing she thought of: she slathered our bare blistering bodies with baking soda, butter, and molasses.

"It probably wasn't the best thing," the hospital nurse said, "but what's done is done." Then she turned to us. "You're two lucky girls, you know that? Those burns could have been a whole lot worse."

We looked at each other and chuckled when she left the room. We sure didn't feel like two lucky girls. We'd take her word for it though. Rather than just sitting around being sad and sore, we let ourselves get a little goofy. Not a good idea. Especially when, in the middle of our fun, I knocked over a drinking glass. Instantly, its smash set off my panic buttons. "Broom!" I cried. "Quick, I need a broom!"

Desperate to quiet me, the nurse fetched me one. "No worries," she said. As fast as I could, I gathered the mess into the dustpan and hurried to the trashcan to hide the evidence. That's when my pink slippers stopped in front of a big pair of black shoes. Tilting my chin up, I found myself looking into the eyes of a great big doctor. At that moment, the dustpan went limp in my hands, dumping all those tiny shards of glass all over his shoes.

"Do you remember that, Mary Lois? I've never been so terrified in my life. I think that was almost worse than the woodshed."

She laughed. "But God was with us. And here we are, all these years later, too stubborn to let another hospital visit spoil our joy."

Two hours of laughter and reminiscing slipped away before I realized what I was doing. Using the upper part of my toes, I was moving my right foot under my left one—and it felt relaxing. Soothing. Was I on to something?

I said good-bye to Mary Lois and kept rubbing.

Thank you, God, for this new relaxation. Please heal me . . .

By the time morning light beamed through my window, my foot actually looked a whole lot straighter. I couldn't stop staring at it.

"Look," I told the nurse. "I've learned how to relax it. I've been rubbing it all night, and it's making a big difference. It's helping."

She studied it closely and stepped back. "Oh, my gosh. It's even straighter than before. And you say you've just been rubbing it?"

"Yeah, rubbing it and praying through the night."

She laughed. "Really? Well, who would have guessed? Hmm, maybe we need to rethink how we do physical therapy around here."

That sounded fantastic. Clearly, the gentle touch had worked wonders compared to all their cramming, jamming, and forcing.

I couldn't wait to go home and show Eddie. As soon as Daddy dropped me off, I went to the living room to say hello. "You've gotta see this," I said, sticking my foot on the couch.

Casually, he turned my way. "That's nice . . ."

"Eddie? Maybe you should call the boys and tell them."

He thought for a second. "Yeah, maybe later."

He hardly showed a spark of emotion, but still, for him, it was something, and my heart warmed. Not only was my foot on the mend, but it gave Eddie a good reason to call the boys. I followed him to the kitchen. "What's this?" I asked. He followed my pointy finger to the stack of envelopes on the counter.

"Bills," he said. "Garretts stopped paying."

"They did *what*? Why did they do that? I'll have to phone Shanda. I'm sure it's just a misunderstanding. She'll straighten it out."

I hadn't talked to Shanda since she visited the hospital with the big-wigs, so I welcomed an opportunity to connect.

"I'm on the mend," I told her. "I'm calling about Garretts' insurance. I see they stopped paying my medical bills."

The instant I said "bills," her tone sounded strained and formal.

"Ema, you've been off work for five months. Your account can't stay active forever."

"What? They can't just cut me off, can they?" I tried to sound calm. "Well, how do we make it active again?"

"You could always come back to work."

I stared at my slightly crooked foot. Well, it *did* look a whole lot better.

"I'm still on crutches," I told her, "but I suppose I could come back to work."

"That would be wonderful," she said. "We'll start you off with just a couple hours. And you can stand at the door and hand out carts like you used to."

That settled it. If I wanted medical coverage, I'd have to go back to work a little sooner. That's what I'd do then. But first, I had a great big fear to face.

Return

September 1993

I arrived at Shanda's office extra early. She already knew my plan. I hobbled behind her along the store's edge. Hopefully nobody would see me. Not yet.

Sweat gathered under my arms as we neared the storage room. *I can do all things through Christ who gives me strength. The Lord is the strength of my life.*

I wanted to reverse my steps and tear out of the building, but if I didn't do this, how in the world would I ever be able to work here again? Whenever I saw ladders these days, whether in stores or at playgrounds, my heart picked up so I could hardly breathe. I'd never had a phobia before, but I'd heard avoidance only makes things worse.

Shanda stopped in front of the big double doors. "You sure you want to do this?"

I nodded. As she swung open the door, I felt that all-too-familiar heat wave.

"You're a brave woman, Ema."

Tell that to my heart, I wanted to say. It pounded so fast I wondered if I'd pass out all over again. Do it, I told myself. *I will lift up my eyes to the hills. Where does my help come from?*

There it was—the ladder ... *My help comes from the Lord, maker of heaven and earth.*

I clenched my jaw so my teeth wouldn't clatter. My body's reaction felt foreign, almost as if my cells remembered what I tried to forget: the jutting boards … the long steel beams … The memories crashed down, only heightening my headache. My eyes traced the underside of the loft and stopped at the gap by the wall. There it was: the likely place where Kyle had seen my dangling arm and hand. The place where he turned on his heel, ran up the ladder, and found my twisted hanging body.

I shivered. How on earth had I survived hanging upside down for two and a half hours by my left foot? It hit me full force: I could have so easily died. Kyle could have missed that stray clothes rack. He could have left it out for somebody else. But no, God directed him to see it so he'd push it into the storage room and rush to help me. Otherwise, I would have been left hanging upside down until Monday morning.

I felt fresh gratitude. This wasn't a room of tragedy. It was a room of deliverance.

Thank you, Jesus, for helping me see it that way.

I walked to my old section smiling. Several coworkers saw me and called out, "Look who's here." Everybody opened their arms and rang in a chorus of joy: "Ema! I can't believe it." "We're sorry this happened." "Are you really coming back to work?" "It's great to see you!"

As Kyle gave me a hug, a simple understanding passed between us. Pulling back, I noticed his eyes looked moist. "Thank you," I told him. "It's good to be here." Then I looked to the others. "I've really missed this place. I missed you guys, my customers, everything."

Shanda didn't need to give me any instructions on how to be a door greeter again. It came back as naturally as chewing a piece of gum — which, incidentally, I had to do for my medicine-induced dry throat.

Maneuvering on crutches felt awkward, so I quickly learned how to move around on just one. I handed out carts, winked at kids, smiled at customers, and made small talk the way I always had. "How's it going?" "I like your earrings." "Isn't it a great day to be alive?" I got so into it that I overlooked my pain and exhaustion. I kept pressing it down.

Two weeks later, it tanked. My foot hurt so much that I had to duck into the restroom and splash water on my face. The shock temporarily distracted me, but it didn't do anything for my pain. I didn't get it. How could it hurt so much even with pain medicine?

As I stood at the door, shifting from leg to leg, Dr. Noll's words echoed in my head like a sentence of doom: "Ema, you're just going to have to learn to live with the pain."

My two-hour shifts soon got switched to four. And a few months later, the four-hour stretches got pushed into six. They didn't just ask me to hand out carts anymore. They had me running all over the place. And since my foot hurt whether I used the crutch or not, I often set it down. Crutch or no crutch, I ended up putting a lot of weight on that bent-over ankle anyway—so what difference did it make?

At home, I'd try rubbing my feet together like I did at the hospital, but this time it wouldn't do anything. My foot wouldn't relax and straighten like before.

God, why isn't it helping anymore?

As much as I tried, the foot wouldn't cooperate. One frustrating night, I dragged myself to the kitchen to grab a snack. That's when I saw a couple envelopes on the counter. Bills. Pulling out one of the statements, my stomach tightened. Insurance had stopped paying again.

When I knocked on Shanda's door, she almost looked like she expected me.

"I don't know what's going on," I said, "but these statements show that Garretts isn't covering my medical bills anymore. Do you know anything about it?"

"Actually, I do. You're only covered for a certain period of time, and it looks like you've reached that point."

"I don't get it. This was a work-related accident. Are they not even going to pay for some of these past tests and treatments? And what about my medications? They aren't cheap."

She shrugged. "Look, I talked to the powers that be, and the long and the short of it is: Garretts isn't liable. That's all I can tell you."

"What do you mean Garretts isn't liable?"

She crossed her arms. "Just what I said. We're not liable."

When I told Eddie, he had his head in a crossword puzzle. "Yeah, they're liable."

"That's not what Shanda just told me. What should we do?"

He filled in a word. "We need to talk to a lawyer."

"Good idea, but who?"

Just then, I noticed several newspapers beside Eddie. The front page on one of them said: "Minnesota's Top 20 Lawyers." Of all things.

"Eddie, did you see what's beside you?"

"Newspapers," he said without looking up.

Snatching the paper, I turned to the appropriate page and randomly picked one. And that's how we ended up in Charlie Bird's office.

Law and Disorder

October 1994

Charlie stood almost eye to eye to my five feet eleven inches. He had an easy smile and sharp blue eyes that looked like they didn't miss a beat.

"Let's hear more about this," he said.

I'd rather eat worms than rehash my accident, but I had no choice. So back to the storage room I went. Back to those products, boxes, Kleenex, and, of course, the heater.

"From what you're saying," Charlie said, "it doesn't sound like their heater had standard safety deflectors. The deflectors direct heat away from people, something that sadly didn't happen in your situation."

"So is Garretts liable?"

"I'd love to work with you," he said. "After you sign a retainer agreement, we can send someone over to Garretts to check it out. But from everything you're telling me, it sounds like we've got ourselves a really strong case."

I pumped his hand. "Thanks, Charlie. I'll give it some serious thought and call you back."

December 1, 1994

After a long, hard day at work, all I wanted to do was go home to my apartment and collapse on my bed like a rag doll. My keys jangled in the lock as I hummed "Joy to the World." But when the door creaked open, something didn't feel quite right.

"Eddie? Are you home?"

I hurried to the bedroom and stopped in my tracks. Boxes lay scattered all over the floor.

"Eddie, what are you doing?"

"I'm packing," he said matter-of-factly. "I'm leaving. Moving into my mother's house."

My heart pounded. "Just like that? No fight, no conversation, nothing?"

He kept his eyes on the boxes. "I'm getting out of here."

I needed air. And time to think. I hurried to the spare bedroom and dove under the covers.

After more than twenty-five years of prayer and this is what it came to? My mind flooded with questions. When did he decide this? *Why* did he decide this? Did he do it because he felt weak or incapable? I'd read books about that.

Right from day one, Eddie had always wanted a certain amount of control. That's why he never let me get my driver's license. I assumed I'd take the test after we got married, but no, Eddie wouldn't hear of it.

"Why not?" I asked. "It would be good for both of us."

But my pleas fell on deaf ears, and he always answered the same: "You've got me. You don't need a license. I can take you wherever you need to go."

Well, if he wanted to make me dependent on him, the accident sure gave him his wish. Apparently, he didn't find driving me around all that it was cracked up to be. Kind of like our marriage. For years, we'd been driving around in circles, going absolutely nowhere. God knew I'd made my share of mistakes. I just wished things had turned out differently.

※

After Eddie moved out, I threw myself into my work, putting everything into it. I loved on the customers — always trying to add that extra spark to their day.

To make life easier, I left the old apartment and moved into a smaller one right across the street from Garretts. It took only a few dozen steps to get to their parking lot.

One day while crossing the street, the unthinkable happened. My left ankle seized up in the middle of the road. Buckling over, I collapsed on the pavement.

"Help!" I screamed, knowing a car could come any second.

Just then, someone honked and hollered, "Ema!"

What? Who was that? Her voice sounded familiar. Lana? Sure enough — of all people.

She rushed over and helped me to my feet. "Let's get you in my car."

Leave it to God to use the same person who didn't drive me home the night of my accident to now pick me up in the middle of the road.

"Need a ride to the hospital?"

I shook my head. "No, thank you. I just need you to take me home."

And I never returned to Garretts again.

Friends and Enemies

January 1995

Concern darkened Dr. Noll's face as he examined me. "The RSD has moved into your ankle again. We need you back on those crutches. I'd also like to give you morphine for the pain."

My left foot pointed more downward and inward than ever, almost in an angry twist. How sad to have been so close to healing, only to end up like this.

As Daddy drove home, he couldn't hide the worry in his eyes. Ever since Eddie stepped out, Daddy stepped up. He reminded me of Moses leading the Israelites out of the desert, that barren land that went on and on. Naturally, I wanted to grumble and complain, but why throw that on Daddy when it would only make things worse?

Whenever I caught myself inwardly complaining, God reminded me to think of something true, lovely, and pure. It wasn't as easy to cast off worry though. How quickly it snuck up like a hungry wolf, especially when I imagined the future.

Sorry, God, I'm worrying again. I know you're trustworthy and you'll always take care of me.

I looked at Daddy. "What are you thinking?"

He took his time answering. "I'm thinking about all the junk you're going through *and* how God must have an extra big plan in all of this."

I knew he was right. God wouldn't take me through the desert without leading me to some kind of promised land. I just hoped I wouldn't have to wander around in the desert for forty years first.

As I waited for my healing, I knew God wanted me to look at the good things in the desert. Daddy was one of those bright spots, a refreshing oasis. Charlie Bird was another.

Thanks to Charlie's legal prowess, Garretts' insurance had started paying again. Charlie confirmed that the heater didn't have safety deflectors, so yes, Garretts was liable.

But the insurance company wasn't willing to accept this without taking action. They kept forcing me to get second opinions—like the one with Dr. Thomas Mazer at the North Pain Institute in Minneapolis.

February 6, 1995

Dr. Mazer bit down on his lip. "Ema, this is quite unfortunate."

I fidgeted with my hands. "What do you mean?"

"Well, if insurance hadn't forced you back to work so fast *and* if you'd stayed off your feet for several months straight, things might have been different. I'm convinced you could have gotten all that RSD worked out of your foot for good."

Instinctively, my fingers reached for my cross necklace. "What are you saying?"

"I'm saying you were almost there, Ema. You just needed to give it more time. All that weight and pressure you've been putting on your foot has spun your RSD into a vicious cycle."

Regret twisted my gut. His words made sense all right, but what could I say?

He shook his head. "I looked at your medical records, and frankly, I'm floored by your epidural. They gave you a whopping dose, didn't they? Two epidurals in one day? Good night."

"They only did it because none of the epidurals worked. I felt *all* the pain in my left leg, and I could move it both times."

His eyes widened. "We're definitely dealing with advanced RSD here. On the bright side, this will all help insurance see that you're a prime candidate for some serious medical treatment."

Then it struck me. "Can *you* help me with this?"

"Wish I could," he said. "But unfortunately, your muscles, tendons, and nerves are far too damaged. I'm very sorry."

March 31, 1995

After I gave the news to Dr. Noll, he sent me to another doctor.

Dr. C. A. Peterson was soft-spoken and kind. He believed with his whole heart and soul he could straighten my crooked left ankle.

"We can fix this. I'd like to do a special procedure that will loosen the buildup around your ankle. Unfortunately, it will involve putting you in a cast for a month. But I think the extra time will make a difference."

"Whatever helps," I told him. Frankly, I'd try anything. I felt like a warm slab of clay in the molding process—except I already felt the fire.

A couple days after the procedure, my good friend Ellie came over to see if she could help.

"I don't want to just sit around and do nothing," I told her. "I need to get my mind off this pressing, itchy cast before it drives me nuts."

She cocked her head. "Need anything from the store?"

"Hmm, maybe some baggy pants to stretch over this beast."

"Okay, let's do it," she said. I loved how Ellie took time out of her busy weekend to help. Another oasis in my desert.

We went to TJ Maxx and soon ended up in different sections. Eventually, I needed to use the restroom. No big deal. How hard could it be?

Then again, what did I know? Let's just say, it didn't take me long to develop fresh empathy for people on crutches. Those long wooden extensions made everything more difficult in those tiny public restroom stalls.

Speaking of stalls. After I flushed, my door wouldn't open. The lock was completely jammed! I pushed, pulled, twisted, or turned, but absolutely nothing happened. The old blue door clanged and banged as I worked to open it, but it refused to cooperate. Great. How long would I be in there before Ellie found me?

As soon as someone entered the restroom, I rattled harder.

"Hey, are you okay in there?" the voice responded.

"Yeah, *I'm* fine. But my door's jammed."

"Oh, dear, I'll see if I can help." She sounded like an older woman, but I'd take help at any age. Together, we pushed, pulled, rattled, and strained.

"Honey, this baby ain't going nowhere," she exclaimed.

I became indignant. "Well, if the door isn't going to budge, I'm coming under!" Without hesitating, I dropped to the floor and stuck my legs under the door.

She gasped. "Ma'am? You're in a cast."

"I know that, but I still need to get out. Do you think you could give me a hand?"

For a second I thought she'd left, but then I felt a cold, clammy hand come down on my leg. "I don't know about this," she said. "I don't want to hurt you."

"Don't worry," I assured her. "Just give me your best pull and we'll get me out of here."

While she grunted and tugged, I did my very best to relax and make it easy. That's when I realized, *Uh-oh. The opening's smaller than I thought.*

"Can you pull any harder? Grab my arms."

"Ah ... I'm really not sure about this." But she pulled on my arms and I started to slide.

"We're almost there," I said. Good thing, because I was getting tired of looking at the ugly old ceiling that needed a new paint job.

Ever so slowly, she slid my body across the cold beige tiles. And joy of joys, I saw her bright smiling face, glowing with relief and perspiration.

Praise God, I was free!

After she pulled me to my feet, we broke into laughter. Ellie walked in with eyes the size of a hoot owl.

"Ellie, I'd like you to meet this really nice woman who saved me." I paused. "What's your name?"

"Alice."

"I'd like you to meet Alice."

Ellie said a quick "hello," then looked at me as she spoke. "It's always an adventure with Ema."

A few days later, I had what you might call a physical therapy adventure. It happened when Dr. Clause assigned me to Vance Wade, the very therapist who made me climb the staircase on crutches after my accident. I couldn't believe it.

"How are you doing?" he said. "We're going to do something to help your circulation." He lifted my leg up and down like a drawbridge. "Don't forget to do this at home."

Maybe in my dreams, I thought.

When I saw him the next week, his eyes flashed with determination. "We need to remove your cast so we can get down to business."

I stared at him. "Really? It's only been two weeks. Dr. Peterson told me I need to keep it on for a month."

He scribbled out a prescription. "No. Here you go. I want you to go downstairs to orthopedics and give this to the receptionist. Someone will take off your cast, then you can come back up for the rest of your therapy."

I didn't say anything to Daddy until we got to the hall. "Since when do therapists write prescriptions?"

Daddy shook his head, frustrated. "I know. Something doesn't sound right."

My foot and leg ached as I hobbled down the hall and stepped in the elevator. Maybe getting my cast removed wasn't such a bad idea.

I got off the elevator and made it to the check-in desk. When my turn came, I smiled at the clerk and gave her my name and birth date. We then followed a nurse to a room where half a dozen other people waited. Dr. Peterson looked up and did a double take. "What are you guys doing here?"

I handed him the prescription. "Vance Wade wants it off."

He frowned. "Please excuse me for a minute." Everybody stared as he stepped out.

When he returned, he tore up my prescription. "The cast stays. See you in two weeks."

What could I say except "thank you" and head back to the elevator. Great. Now we had to face our favorite therapist and finish my appointment.

At least when we stepped in the elevator, God gave me some giggly girls to make me smile.

"Have a nice day," I told them as I stepped off.

Most people would have loved to get their cast off early, but I had something else in mind — a future goal. I wanted a better, straighter foot, not just a little temporary relief. If wearing the cast longer would make things better in the long run, well, of course I'd keep it on.

Vance shook his head when we stepped back into the physical therapy examination room. "Now look what you've done. I can't help you anymore. My hands are tied."

Deflated, I couldn't hobble out of there fast enough.

"Well, that was really something," my dad said in the hallway.

"You think that's bad," I said, "you should have heard him after the accident when they first put me on crutches."

"That guy has an attitude," he said. "If I was you, I'd switch therapists. You have that right, you know."

I breathed deeply, knowing what I wanted to do. And let me tell you: the idea of not needing to deal with him anymore felt really good.

A few days later, my cousins Jane, Joyce, Daisy, and Myrna came over to visit.

"We're going to distract you from your pain," Jane said. She's the oldest. She took all of us on a trip down memory lane. One memory led to another, and before I knew it, I was a fire hose of old stories. They sped through my mind like videos, sending me running across grassy farm fields where it all began with my brothers and sisters in Traer, Iowa.

After Mom hung her laundry outside, she pulled out a chair and watched us kids play.

One day she said, "It's time. I'm going to the hospital to bring us home a new baby." I was so excited I thought I'd burst. Every day, I bugged Grandma Reeves. "Is it time yet? When's she coming home with the baby?"

"Soon," Grandma said. "You'll know it's time when you hear me shout for you in the field."

True to her word, she hollered into the trees, "Baby's home!" And my little legs couldn't carry me fast enough.

When Mom placed that little bundle on the table and peeled back the coverings, I almost forgot to breathe. Heaven had come down. "That's *my* baby," I said. And I staked my claims on little Murray, holding him, loving him, holding his bottle.

Somehow that led us to talk about the next place where I lived: at the milking farm with all the cows. Daddy always dreamed of having cows, so when I turned eight, we moved to a beautiful house in Wisconsin. It had seven rooms and a big red barn. Plenty of space for the cousins to visit.

Before my cousin Linda stayed with us, she never knew where milk came from. That first time she watched Daddy milking the cows, her eyes grew as wide as saucers. She crossed her arms in front of her chest. "That's disgusting! I'm never drinking that stuff ever again. Only the kind that comes from the store."

Mom kept her cool because she had an idea. When Linda wasn't looking, Mom switched bottles. She filled the store-bought one with the fresh stuff. "Taste any better?" she asked.

Linda's small sips turned to big gulps. "Oh, much better. Thank you, Auntie."

The cousins laughed, recalling other details. Like how my brothers knew all the cows by name.

"Oh, remember your dad's snow scoop?" Joyce said.

How could anybody forget? We had a mile-long driveway which meant, when the snow piled high, we really didn't have a way to get around it. But trust Daddy to dream up a plan. He stuck the old snow scoop on the front of the tractor and scooped all six of us kids into it. He threw an army blanket over us and carried us down the driveway so we could catch the school bus. And we never missed a day.

Man, we loved that dream home. But when Grandpa McKinley got sick two years later, Daddy wanted to move back to Iowa and help him out. That's how we ended up at the house on the hill.

"That house was my favorite," Daisy said.

"Yeah, great family reunions up there," Jane said. "We'd drive up that big hill and one of us would get out and lift the gate."

"That house had the most beautiful timber," I said.

Joyce nodded. "And the most beautiful horses to ride in the field."

I got dreamy as I spoke. "There's just something about running wild 'n' free and letting the breeze catch your hair."

The room got quiet and I felt their eyes on my cast.

"How's it feel?" Joyce asked.

"Umm, horrible."

She sighed. "Will you give us a call when it comes off?"

"You bet," I said. "I'll probably want to throw a party."

When the big day finally came, Dr. Peterson looked anxious to get it off. "You're a patient woman, Ema. But I'm sure it will be worth the wait. Your foot and ankle should look a whole lot straighter."

My heart picked up as the circular saw bit into the plaster.

"Here goes," he said. And I held my breath as he peeled back the thick, dusty layers.

Then our hearts stopped. Right before our eyes, my foot, still red and puffy, slid right back into its same old crooked position.

Hot Seat

July 1995

The failed procedure skyrocketed my pain something terrible. I felt it as I stepped into Charlie Bird's office, practically hanging off my crutches.

He swung open the door to his office. "Thanks for coming on such short notice. Come in. Have a seat."

"You sounded pretty serious on the phone," I said. "I hope I'm not in trouble."

He ran a hand through his hair. "Ema, your insurance is being difficult."

"What else is new?"

"I mean *extra* difficult. They don't think you're getting better fast enough."

"Well, tell them I'll try harder."

"Ema, they want to enroll you in a special program, and they can discontinue paying your claims if you don't comply."

My heart raced. "They could do that?"

He nodded.

"Well, what do they want me to do?" I asked.

"They want to send you to a pain management clinic. They say the pain's all in your head. They often do this kind of thing. It's their attempt to get out of paying."

"Can't you do something? I mean, what do they know about my pain? Sure it's in my head. You can tell them I've had a nonstop migraine ever since the accident. And now I have hearing problems. The doctors say I've lost close to 60 percent of my hearing. Of course, insurance says I can't prove it wasn't like that all along, because I didn't take a hearing test before the accident." I looked straight at him. "Where exactly is this program?"

He cleared his throat. "It's at Generose."

My heart sank. Everyone knew what that hospital building was known for. "They want to stick me in the psych ward? You've got to be kidding."

"Wish I was."

"Well, what's it about?"

"They sent us a video. Why don't we watch it and go from there." He aimed the remote at the television and lively music filled the air. People did jumping jacks and all kinds of rigorous exercises. Impossible exercises for someone like me. How could any of this possibly help me manage my pain?

Charlie stopped the video, and my eyes pleaded with him. "There's no way I could handle a program like that. Either emotionally or physically."

"Ema, you don't have a choice. If you want insurance to pay your medical expenses, you've got to go through this pain management program."

"Couldn't we educate them about RSD? Maybe show them a doctor's note or something . . . I don't know." I tried to swallow as he shook his head. "How long will it last?"

"It's a six-week inpatient program."

"Inpatient?" My stomach tightened. "Charlie, they don't have a clue about my situation."

"You're right, they don't, and I'm sorry about that." He rose to his feet. "They want you to start immediately."

"So that's it then?"

He nodded. "I'm afraid so."

As I packed my suitcase, I thought of Eddie packing his boxes and walking out of my life forever. What was he doing now? Enjoying one of his mother's home-cooked meals probably. Chicken and dumplings or lasagna—who knows?

Houses, stores, and buildings blurred beneath my tears as Daddy drove me to the pain management clinic.

"Let's pray," he said. *"Father God, we thank you for loving us in every situation. We need your help and direction as Ema goes into this program. Help her feel how close you are. Help her trust you and see you at work in a personal way. Thank you that you work all things together for our good. In Jesus' name. Amen."*

He pulled up to a tall brick building that looked more like a prison than a branch of a hospital. A prison they'd sentenced me to for all the wrong reasons.

A nurse smiled at us in the entryway. "Welcome," she said. "My name's Gwen. You have a few minutes to visit before we need to move on. But I should probably let you know that once you're admitted, you can't have any calls or visitors for the first three days."

A young man with oily black hair mumbled to himself as he passed. Was this really happening?

Daddy dropped my suitcase, making me jump. "Sorry," he said. And I fell into his embrace.

We talked for another minute before Gwen walked over. "Are you ready for me to take you around?"

If I wasn't mistaken, Daddy's eyes looked red. Clearly, he'd trade spots with me in a heartbeat. "God will take care of you, Ema. I love you."

Don't turn around, I told myself as I followed the nurse. I knew what would happen if I did. The floodgates would break loose and I'd look like a blubbering idiot.

Gwen led me to a little room with a big desk, and I signed paper after paper, signing my life away.

Then she took me down a hall with a black metal rail on both sides and an intercom on the middle of the wall, right beside the telephone I couldn't use for the next three days.

Lord, keep me strong.

We rounded a corner and stopped at the end of a second hallway.

"Here we are," Gwen said. "Welcome to your room."

She opened the door and I looked around at the two gray chairs, night table, and off-white bed, my mansion for the next six weeks.

"Just drop off your stuff," she said. "We need to get going because they're waiting for you in the conference room."

"They're waiting? Who's waiting?"

"Oh, the staff. They're waiting to give you the hot seat."

"The what seat?"

She gave a suppressed chuckle as she closed the door. "The hot seat is standard procedure for all new patients. You sit at a long table with doctors, nurses, therapists, and teachers, and they give you the rundown on the rules and regulations."

"Sounds interesting," I said. In other words, it sounded horrible. My mind spun as I hurried to keep her pace.

"Here we are," she said, stopping in front of a door.

The mesh of voices quieted when she opened it, and everyone looked at me, studying the new patient.

"Right over there," Gwen said, nodding at the only chair available. I slipped in quickly, but also tried to be extra careful as I stuck my crutches under the table. It would have been horrible to poke a leg and somehow ruffle someone's feathers before we even started.

"Hello, Ema. I'm Dr. Dylan Hayze," a silver-haired man said. "Welcome to our program."

I returned his smile. But as I looked around the table, my heart suddenly froze—

Vance Wade!

Breathe, I told myself. What in the world? I knew he worked at that other hospital, but here too? A heavy dread crept over me, but I tried to look calm and natural. The last thing I wanted was to fall apart and look like I actually belonged here.

Dr. Hayze straightened his notes. "As you know, Ema, every program has its own set of rules and regulations. We're no exception. We expect you to be on time for all your classes. All designated exercises and learning sessions are for your own good. We don't want any complaining, and we don't want any switching of instructors or therapists."

My heart sank as his words echoed in my head. His comment could only mean one thing: Vance had told them about me switching at the hospital. Great. I squeezed my hands under the table. So much for starting off on the right foot. I was already in trouble. I waited for a chance to explain, but they talked for forty-five minutes with no openings.

Hands under his chin, Dr. Hayze grinned as he shared his concluding remark: "We trust your time here will be most productive and beneficial."

I couldn't grab my crutches and get out of there fast enough. I needed air.

"You okay?" Gwen said in the hallway.

"Sure. Other than the fact I feel judged, voiceless, and extremely uncomfortable."

She drew in a breath. "Well, it *is* called the hot seat, after all. I'm sorry you felt that way though. Come. Let's take you to the cafeteria."

The more I stepped closer, the more I smelled something like sizzling pieces of bacon. We rounded a corner and I followed her through a wide set of double doors that opened to a huge cafeteria. I felt like I'd entered a whole new atmosphere that felt a whole lot less hospital-like. Potted plants, big picture windows with welcoming splashes of light, and the beautiful sound of voices talking all at once.

"There's your spot," Gwen said, pointing to a rectangular table where a couple ladies looked up.

"Hi, I'm Mary-Beth," the one with the short hair said. "And this is Viola."

I nodded. "Great to meet you. I'm Ema. What's on the menu?"

Viola rolled her eyes. "Cold cuts, pork and beans."

So much for sizzling bacon, except for the bits in the beans. Looking down I noticed Viola had a sketchpad against her chair.

"Are you an artist?" I asked.

"I guess," she said, shrugging. "I love drawing."

"Oh, don't let her modesty fool ya," Mary-Beth said. "She's an artist and she's good."

"I love art," I told her, "and all things creative. Back when I ran a home day care, I used to paint cute pictures all over my walls. I also used art as a teaching tool."

"Interesting," she said. "How did you do that?"

"I kept it simple. At mealtimes I used special markers to draw faces on the kids' fruit. I also arranged the veggies on their plates to look like characters. Anything to get the kids to eat healthy. Oh, and I drew pictures of talking vegetables and hung them on the wall so I could read them to the kids. The apple said, 'I'm delicious,' and the green bean said, 'I like you.' That kind of thing."

Mary-Beth set down her water. "Did it work?"

"Mostly. One time a little girl jumped out of her chair and shook her finger at my green bean, shouting, 'Well, I don't like *you*!' Other than that it worked, I suppose."

"That's hysterical," Viola said. "Sounds like you ran a fun day care."

I slopped some beans on my plate. "We were the only day care in town that integrated disabled children. Everybody loved it because we all learned from each other."

"Cool," Mary-Beth said. "Have you always been interested in helping handicapped children?"

I sat back dreamily. "For as far back as I can remember. My mom's sister, my Aunt Eva Mae, got a fever when she was five. She never grew up physically or mentally. She stayed like a little girl, and they always let me take care of her. At family reunions, I enjoyed pushing her wheelchair around so she could visit everybody. What a sweetheart. My mom made matching clothes for Aunt Eva Mae and her doll. I'd take her out to the big row of trees and we'd laugh 'til our sides hurt."

"Sounds like you had a perfect childhood," Mary-Beth said.

I snickered. "It was good, but not perfect. I have my regrets like everybody else."

"If anybody knows about regrets," Mary-Beth said, "I do."

Viola looked at her curiously. "Oh, yeah? Like what?"

Mary-Beth stabbed her fork into a slice of ham. "I'll tell you after Ema shares first."

"Well, it isn't a really big deal," I said, "but I regret that I wasn't allowed to do sports. My siblings and I weren't allowed to get involved outside of gym class. That was really hard for me because I excelled at things like jumping hurdles, pole-vaulting, shot-putting, gymnastics, softball—basically, all of it. My teachers and friends urged me to play, but Mom didn't drive and Daddy ran the farm, so ... it was just one of those things."

Viola frowned. "That's too bad. What was your favorite sport?"

I laughed. "Probably softball."

"What's so funny?" Mary-Beth said.

"Oh, just an old memory."

"Must be a good one," she said.

"Well, I don't know if you'd call it that," I said. "One time in gym class, I hit the ball so hard that it went way past the field and ended up smashing into someone's kitchen window. It definitely wasn't funny at the time, especially when my gym teacher made me knock on the lady's door and tell her I'd pay for it. She was a hoot, that woman.

She said, 'No way, young lady. Anybody who can hit a ball that far shouldn't have to pay for anybody's window.'"

Viola shook her head. "I'd be lucky if I hit the ball in the first place."

"My big regret is being here," Mary-Beth said, pushing away her plate. "This place is seriously driving me crazy."

I tried not to laugh at the irony. "We'll make it," I assured them. "God will give us the strength."

It's a good thing I didn't know what awaited me.

Push and Shove

When I walked into the big physical therapy room, I felt like I'd stepped into Charlie's video — except nobody could push the "stop" button.

People were gathered around the instructor doing jumping jacks. Others pumped weights at the side and stretched on mats.

A vanilla-skinned woman walked over. "Hi, are you Ema Lano?"

"Yup, that's me."

Her skinny eyebrows went up. "Good. We've assigned you your own activity supervisor. I think you may have met him at your preliminary meeting. Here he comes. This is Vance Wade."

For a second I forgot to breathe.

"Good morning, Ema," Vance said. "Shall we start off with some floor exercises? Maybe some sit-ups."

Lord, have mercy . . .

Trying not to look like a glazed-over zombie, I dropped my crutches to lower myself to the mat. Perhaps he'd give me a hand? Or not. Instead, he watched as I teetered back and forth until I lost my balance and fell *splat* on the mat.

"I'll count for you," he said.

"Thanks." I heaved my body up and down to the monotone sound of his voice: "One steamboat, two steamboat . . ." He took it to ten. "Now straighten your legs and keep 'em straight. I want you to lift one foot, then the other."

Did he even have a clue what he was asking me to do? I could move my right leg, no problem, but my left leg didn't want to be messed with.

"Mind over matter," he said. "Come on, you can do this. Kick it out and touch the ceiling." Determined to show my willingness, I did what he asked. Pain shot clear up to my knee.

He gave a clap with his hands. "Good. Now on your feet."

Rolling to my left side, I set my right foot on the floor and anchored myself with the crutch for leverage. I tried to pull up my body. It trembled and teetered, but I somehow managed to stand.

If Vance could have known the kind of strength it took for me to do this, he would have applauded, but instead he turned on his heel and announced, "Time for the weights."

Weights? I looked at the wall and the long line of tables with bins on them.

"I want you to pick up a basket, grab an item from each bin, and drop the item in the basket. Then I want you to walk to the other side, remove your items, and walk back here with your empty basket. *Comprendre?*"

I *comprendoed*, but how in the world did he expect me to pull that off on a pair of crutches?

Determined to give it my best, I wedged my crutches under my arms and used my right hand to grab a basket. It dangled beside my crutch, and I had to set it down so I could reach in the bin for my first item, a beanbag. From the next bin I retrieved a heavy ball, and from the third, a horseshoe. The heavier my basket became, the more my crutches dug into my arms. I kept pushing myself. Meanwhile, Vance whistled, stealing glances at his watch. "I'd like you to do it five times," he said.

If he saw the pain in my face, he didn't let on. I wondered how many times he'd make me repeat this before I collapsed.

After three times, I paused to take a breath. "Is this good enough?"

He shook his head. "Two more times."

My movements became slower, stiffer, and my prayers went right along with them.

Lord, please help.

When I dropped the last item into the bin and showed him my empty basket, he didn't smile or blink. He just asked me, "Are you ready for jumping jacks?"

I must have turned red.

"On second thought," he said, "let's save the fun stuff for later."

Two weeks into the program, Vance approached me in the PT room with a three-pronged cane walker. "Time to lose the crutches," he said.

My breath caught in my throat as I looked at my crooked foot. It had swelled up because I pushed myself too hard. But what would happen if I refused? Would he kick me out of the program? That sure sounded tempting—except I needed insurance to pay my medical bills.

"I can't walk on this foot," I said helplessly.

"Oh, really?" He seemed surprised by my boldness. "Ema, don't tell me you're going to quit before you even try?"

"Please ... you don't know what you're asking. You don't understand RSD."

He crossed his arms. "I understand more than you think. Here's what I want you to do. I want you to hand me your crutches. Then I want you to take one step at a time."

He didn't get it. Every time I moved, I pressed all my weight onto those crutches. My foot hurt so much that I was practically hanging on them, letting them dig into my arms—and he wanted me to put all my weight onto a cane walker?

His eyes bore into me with determination.

Jesus, help me ...

I quietly handed him my crutches.

"Good," he said. "Now hold the cane in the palm of your hand like this." I did what he asked and he gave me a quick nod. "Okay, now keep moving."

Leaning in, I willed myself forward. "Ah ..." The pain shot up from my foot to my hip. "Please," I begged.

"You can do it. Step together step."

Goodness, he sounded like that exercise guru Richard Simmons. My cane walker felt like it was bruising my hand as I took another step. And why did he have to grip my crutches so tight? Did he think I was going to steal them?

I could feel people watching, but I hurt too much to care. I pressed down on that crooked foot, feeling all my weight on my ankle. I hated to think about the damage I was causing.

"Keep going," he said. "We're going to walk you around the corner." Pain escalated with each step. Where was he taking me?

He turned toward a storage room, and I got a bad feeling as he whistled and led the way inside. Then, as if I wasn't even there, he opened a locker and threw in my crutches!

Anger burned in my throat.

"It's dinnertime," he said, "so we're going to have you walk to the cafeteria."

I stared at him blankly. "With the cane walker?"

When he nodded, I knew it wouldn't do any good to argue. I wiped my sweaty hand on my pants, planted it on the cane walker, and battled my way down the hall.

When Mary-Beth and Viola saw me, concern darkened their faces. I don't know how many steps I took before it happened. The cane walker slid out from under my hand, and I collapsed in a heap.

"Stay back," Vance ordered as they rushed over to help. "Ema needs to get up on her own."

I struggled to reach for my cane walker.

"We can help her," Mary-Beth insisted.

Vance waved them off. "No, thanks. You go on ahead to the cafeteria. Ema will be there shortly."

Lord, I'm still asking for help.

I grabbed my cane walker and stood it upright. Jerking back and forth, I somehow managed to pull myself back up while Vance clasped his hands, pleased. "See, that wasn't so bad. Just a few more steps and you'll be eating macaroni and cheese."

But every step slipped me further away from my appetite. And by the time I dropped into my chair between Mary-Beth and Viola, I didn't even want to be there.

Mary-Beth shook her head. "I can't believe he switched you to a cane walker. I mean, look at your foot. It looks like you just came out of surgery."

"It's crazy," Viola agreed. "And Vance wouldn't even let us help you. I felt so helpless."

"Show her your drawing," Mary-Beth said. "Viola just did a quick caricature."

My new artist friend opened her sketchpad to a goofy-looking picture of Vance doing jumping jacks.

"It's for you," Mary-Beth said.

"You guys …" I was laughing in spite of everything. It was just a picture, but it changed the tone for our meal and lightened us up. It sure felt good just to be listened to and understood.

It wasn't until we finished our food and got ready to leave that I realized the nurse hadn't stopped by to give me my pills. Strange. They were always so good about it. Did she forget?

"I need to check out something at the nurses' station," I told my friends.

"We'll help you get there," Viola said.

"Thanks, but I probably need to get used to this thing by myself now." So off I went, slowly, stiffly, painfully, from the warm feel of the cafeteria to the cold, sterile nurses' station.

Catching my breath, I leaned over the counter and managed to half smile at the nurse. "Hi, I'm Ema Lano. They didn't give me my medicine tonight."

Frowning, the nurse thumbed through her paperwork until she found my name. Then she poked her finger on it. "Ema Lano. It says they took you off."

"What?" I said. "They took me off my medications? Really? Nobody said anything."

She shrugged. "All I know is what it says. Can I help you with anything else?"

"No, thanks. I don't think so." And I turned and headed for my room.

Emergency Code

Around noon the next day, my stomach felt queasy. What had I eaten? By midafternoon, I felt hot, and by dinnertime, my teeth clattered.

Father, I'm sick and weak.

Mary-Beth knocked on my door. "Ready for grub?" Taking one look at me, she backed away. "Ema ... you need a nurse."

When Gwen stepped in, her eyebrows shot up. "My word! You look sick as a dog. Must be the flu. One of the other nurses has it. Hang in there. I'll keep checking on you."

While my friends shoveled down meat loaf and rice in the cafeteria, I shook and vomited like nobody's business. I would have called the nurse except she already knew how sick I was.

Lord, I feel like I'm fading ...

I didn't have the strength to make it to the bathroom, so I had no choice but to stay in bed. Vomit and sweat covered my sheets and clothing, but I was too sick to care. Sick and going down faster than a coffin. My whole body felt poisoned.

Mary-Beth poked in after dinner and ran out, hollering for help.

Gwen stepped in and I saw it on her face. Panic. I only heard two words. "Emergency code."

In the next half hour, my room became a sea of doctors, nurses, and equipment. I heard someone say they needed to pull a doctor out of surgery—fast. Time was of the essence and they needed more help.

"You poor thing," one of the nurses said. "You're as hot as an oven."

I groaned. "Please don't take off my covers. I'm freezing." But it didn't matter what I wanted because about every hour they had to flip off my sheets to draw blood from my arm. And when they did it, ice raged in my bones.

I was in and out of it, but somewhat aware of their chatter. It rang with desperate urgency. I heard phrases like "drug withdrawal" and "fatal," and I suddenly understood the magnitude of my situation. I knew with ugly certainty something I wished I didn't: my life was in danger.

I talked to Jesus in fits and starts. Told him how much I loved him, how much I needed to feel him close. Sometimes I had no words, only a deep sense of his presence and a sad awareness of my pain. I didn't know what the doctors and nurses were doing, but on some strange level I knew who was in charge. The Great Physician. Still, I couldn't help but ask the Lord, *Why is this happening?*

A nurse dabbed my forehead with a terry cloth towel. "Your friends are outside the door." She swung it open and sure enough, there they were—the whole big group of them, clumped like raisins: Mary-Beth, Viola, and five or six others. They camped outside my door the whole night—worrying, praying, and keeping a silent vigil.

The doctors and nurses said something about my heart being in bad shape. I didn't know about that, but at least God gave me a few good friends who knew how to reach it. They were like Jesus with skin on, and they didn't want me to suffer alone.

I too kept a silent vigil—under my shaking sheets. As the sweat dripped down, the prayers poured out.

Jesus, please don't let me die ...

The Stairs

I spent the next two days shaking and sweating in bed, thanking God for sparing my life. "For you, LORD, have delivered me from death, my eyes from tears, my feet from stumbling, that I may walk before the LORD in the land of the living" (Psalm 116:8 – 9).

I guess we have more work to do, don't we, God? I don't know what you're trying to teach me, but could I possibly learn it some other way? Maybe from a good book or something?

After everything that happened, you'd think Vance Wade would take it easy on me. But nothing could have been further from the truth. Less than a week after I recovered, we had a serious run-in. I'd just come from watching people play volleyball downstairs, and I felt pretty good because I'd encouraged a young guy to let go of his anger. And boy, did he let it go. I'd never seen someone hit the volleyball so hard. And smile so big afterward. I hadn't stopped smiling myself— until Vance cornered me in front of the elevator.

"No more elevators," he said, stretching out his arm. "From now on, you're taking the stairs."

The stairs? Had I heard correctly? I could tell from the look on my friends' faces that I had. Twenty feet away, Mary-Beth, Viola, and a few others stood at the bottom of the stairs, watching and listening in amazement. We'd just been together, so we'd planned to meet each other at the top.

My heart pounded. Not only did my foot and leg ache, but the rest of me ached as well. After all, I was still weak from the drug withdrawal. How could Vance expect me to climb all twelve stairs with a lousy cane walker?

"I don't have the strength," I told him. "Please let me take the elevator like I normally do."

He shook his head. "I'm sorry, but we need you to take the stairs."

Every ounce of my hurting flesh wanted to refuse, but how could I? For the last several weeks, I'd gone out of my way to encourage and motivate my friends, who now stood watching. Over and over I'd told them, "If we only push through ... If we only do what they tell us to and give it our best, we might actually learn something valuable in the end — something that will make a difference in the long run."

My words seemed to mock me as my peers slowly, somberly stepped up the stairs ahead of me. Again, I didn't see any way to get around this. I was stuck. So I took a deep breath and before I could talk myself out of it, I let go of my cane walker and started my way up. My heart drummed wildly against my chest as I grabbed the railing and, inch by inch, pulled myself up those steep, cold stairs.

I could only imagine what my friends were thinking: how could Vance be so cruel?

When my foot finally touched the top, Mary-Beth wiped her eyes and opened her arms to hug me. Then suddenly she stopped. I think we both remembered the rule at the same time: no hugs.

Back in my room, I cried out to Jesus.

Where are those strong, warm arms of yours? I need to feel them right now. I need to know you'll never turn away from my hugs. And please, I beg you, can I be done with this place?

A few days later, Gwen stopped me in the hallway. "Hi, Ema. We need to talk."

Uh oh. The last time I heard those words, they came from Charlie when he told me I had to go to this program in the first place.

I followed her into a small office beside the nurses' station and tried to relax as she closed the door.

"You'll be glad to know we had a special staff meeting about you."

"What kind of a meeting?"

"I'll be straight with you," she said. "Almost everybody agrees that it makes sense to dismiss you early from the program. You don't need to stay these last couple weeks. This program really wasn't for you."

I didn't know what to say. I probably should have hollered and cheered, but somehow I felt too burned and cheated. It took them four long weeks to come to this?

Gwen shifted on her feet. "If you're okay with it, we'd like to keep your send-off on the simple side. We can meet in the smaller room with no patients present. It'll be just you, me, and Tracy, the insurance representative."

Just hearing the word "insurance" made me cringe. At least my final meeting would be short. Usually their meetings took place in one of the larger classrooms so the other patients could attend and add their two cents if they wanted. I liked those meetings and usually left on cloud nine. When the staff asked the departing person, "What did you get out of the program?" I heard answers that would stay with me forever: "I would never have made it through if it wasn't for Ema Lano. So many times I wanted to quit, but Ema always encouraged me to keep going and give it my best."

As soon as we all arrived for my closing meeting, Gwen got right down to business. "I know you've had quite the time here, Ema, but we still have a couple questions to ask. For one, what did you learn from the program?"

My heart picked up. As much as I had tried to rehearse an answer, I still didn't know what to say. I knew I couldn't lie, but I also didn't want to leave the place on a sour note. *Oh, Lord, please fill my mouth* ... Looking them in the eyes, I felt fresh confidence.

"I learned that I'm much stronger than I thought I was." There, I'd said it. Simple, honest, right, and it seemed to satisfy them.

Thank you, Lord.

Oh, my goodness—something dawned on me: if someone had told me a year ago that I'd end up in a pain management program in a psych ward, I probably would have had a panic attack on the spot.

The insurance representative scribbled something in her notebook as Gwen jumped into her next question: "What did you *not* like about the program?"

Oh, boy. I knew what I *wanted* to say, but how could I say it? And if I didn't say it, I might never have another chance to say it. I took a deep breath. "Well, I don't like how I almost had to die in order to learn my lessons."

The tick of the clock on the wall got louder. Gwen didn't look surprised by my answer. When it came right down to it, why should she be? She knew full well I was referring to the drug withdrawal. On top of that, by constantly pushing me, they'd probably made my foot much worse. All that extra weight, motion, and pressure had surely taken a toll. The pain now stretched clear up to my calf, which looked redder and more swollen than ever.

It felt good to answer their questions, to share what should have been obvious all along: I didn't belong in their program.

As the meeting drew to a close, I actually felt lighter. Like I'd tapped into some new kind of strength that I didn't know I had. A strength I could maybe use in the days ahead.

If only it could have been that easy.

Starting Over

As a welcome-home gift after the pain clinic, I found divorce papers in the mail. So this was it. We were done. I was no longer a Lano, but back to being Ema McKinley. My fingers trembled as I riffled through the pages. Seeing Eddie's signature on something so official brought me back to our wedding certificate.

Sadly, we never did have a marriage. In twenty-six years, we never figured out what it meant to be husband and wife. But through all that time, I never stopped trying, hoping, and praying. The boys saw everything I went through and how I never gave up. That had to count for something, right? I hoped it did.

All those years I'd prayed, *God, please change Eddie.* And now I could see God instead changed *me.* He taught me how to hold on to him and pray Psalm 51:10 right along with David:

"Create in me a pure heart, O God, and renew a steadfast spirit within me."

Out of obedience, I gave God thanks as I prayed this verse.

Thank you, Lord, for using the tough stuff with Eddie to teach me perseverance through this RSD.

※

A couple days after I opened the divorce papers, I sat down to write a poem about the goodness of God. But I didn't get very far before the phone rang.

"Guess what?" Jason said. "Tara's expecting."

I clasped my hands to my chest. "When's she due?"

"The second week in April."

"Oh, Jason. You don't know how much I've been thinking and praying about this."

He chuckled. "I have a pretty good idea."

After I got off the phone, I stepped outside into the sun. I loved the apartment's grassy area where I could recline on a blanket and have quiet times with Jesus.

A short slender mother with her little girl walked by and I smiled at them. "Nice day, isn't it?"

"Perfect," the woman said.

The little girl hid behind her mother, nervous of strangers. Somehow she reminded me of a little girl I met when I was seven.

I'd tagged along with Daddy to visit one of his new friends. The tall, easygoing man had a five-year-old daughter who wouldn't let go of his leg, not even for a second. She clung like a barnacle on a rock while her dad gave us a helpless shrug. "She's scared silly of people. We can't even send her to school. We tried several times, but it never worked. She always throws such a big fit that they end up sending her home."

Something came over me, and I desperately wanted to help. I inched closer and gave the little girl a smile as I pointed out her back window. "Hey, look at those fun-looking swings." When her fingers loosened their grip, I kept going. "I'll bet you know how to pump really, really high."

With that, she pulled out from behind her dad's pant leg and gave me a serious nod.

"Great," I said. "I like pumping too. And I can do some *really* cool stuff when I jump. Wanna see?"

She nodded.

"Okay then," I said. "Let's go. I'll race ya to the swings!"

And off she flew without looking back.

When we got to the car, Daddy beamed proud. "Do you want to know what that little girl's father just told me? He told me his little girl has never in her life trusted a stranger before. You were the very first one. *You*, wee Ema, have a very special gift."

My heart felt like a flying kite. Between that incident with the little girl and other times when I'd helped with Murray and Aunt Eva Mae, I knew more than anything what I wanted to do: I wanted to help others.

So at family reunions I began to take people's crying babies and rock them to sleep. Armed with love and peace, I ached to make a difference. And boy, did the desire run deep. It felt so simple.

Back when the world seemed so fixable.

Back to the Pit

A week and a half after my early release from the pain management clinic, Charlie gave me a call. "I don't know how to tell you this," he said.

"Just spit it out, Charlie."

I lowered myself onto a kitchen chair as he spoke. "Insurance wants you back in the pain management clinic—this time as an outpatient."

My head spun and my hand went to my mouth. No absolute way. This was beyond crazy. It was flat out wrong. The staff themselves had admitted I didn't belong in their program. For goodness' sake, they'd dismissed me early. How on earth could they force me back?

"Are you okay?"

"I don't know," I told him. And I really didn't. This wasn't Charlie's fault, but it seemed ridiculous that he couldn't do anything. I knew better than to push him though. It wouldn't do any good. Just like it wouldn't do Charlie any good to push the insurance company. By this time, we all knew who we were dealing with—and this was all just part of the insurance game. They'd keep pushing and looking for loopholes 'til they found them, and they wouldn't stop until I waved my little white flag in surrender. Well, if they thought I'd give up, they were flat-out wrong, because more than ever, I needed them to cover my medical bills. So if they wanted me to play by their rules, fine. But one way or another, God would be with me and help me face the worst.

When I returned to the pain management clinic, Vance Wade glanced up from the baskets, looking entirely too happy to see me.

I didn't say a word as I wobbled through his exercises with my cane walker. I didn't spill a single feeling about my pain. Didn't want to give him the satisfaction. Instead, I saved my sobs for the restroom. Locking myself in, I buried my face in my hands.

God, please help me.

Just a few words, but he heard them loud and clear—and he reminded me that the enemy wanted to use my pain. Wanted to make me feel distant from my Savior at a time when I needed him most. This insight made me want to stir up my faith even more. I let the words from Psalm 34:18 slip out of my lips: "The LORD is close to the brokenhearted and saves those who are crushed in spirit."

Lord, I'm brokenhearted. Please stay close to me. I'm crushed deeply in my spirit. Please rescue me.

As Daddy helped me get in the car to go home, I didn't look back at the pain management clinic. I didn't tell him how the RSD had sunk its teeth even deeper into my muscles, joints, and nerves. Nor did I tell him how angry I felt. I wrestled with a kaleidoscope of questions and fears. How could the insurance company have done this to me?

My knees hurt and my head pounded the whole ride home. What if they tried to force me to go back? Could they do it again? I wouldn't put it past them. But I knew one thing for sure: I couldn't do it anymore. My body simply wouldn't let me.

Daddy parked in front of my apartment. "Are you sick?"

"I'll be fine."

I felt like an old woman with her guardian Daddy hovering over her. Shouldn't it have been the other way around—me helping him?

I sighed. At least one of us was healthy, *thank you, Lord.* Back when Mom was alive, Daddy had battled cancer twice—and here he was, pouring himself out for me.

He helped me into my apartment and gave me a gentle hug. When he pulled back, I thanked him, gave him a quick wave, and closed the door behind me.

All I wanted to do was collapse on my bed and fall asleep. I tried, but I just couldn't get comfortable. I couldn't escape the pain that pulsed up my arms and legs, invading muscles and tendons I didn't even know I had. What was happening to me?

Tired of twisting and turning, I grabbed my crutches and dragged myself to the living room. At least I could sit on my plush blue chair. Then again, maybe I couldn't. My knees and the back of my legs hurt too much to sit there.

Rocking to my feet, I grabbed my crutches and a pillow and worked my way to the kitchen. If my bed and living room chair wouldn't work for me, well, maybe I'd try something firmer.

Out of sheer exhaustion, my upper body collapsed on my stove. I felt like a big slab of clay smacked on a kiln. From the top of my burners I prayed, *Oh, God, please give me rest. Even just a little.*

Reality Check

October 1995

"It doesn't look good," Dr. Noll said, shaking his head. "The RSD has moved into your left knee, arms, hands, and shoulders."

For all the throbbing, burning, and aching, I shouldn't have been surprised.

He folded his hands. "It's been two and a half years since your accident. We've given you several types of medicine, including morphine—which reminds me: I talked to Dr. Clause. With your new level of pain, we want to put you back on."

"Okay," I said weakly. "Whatever you think."

Whenever I heard a doctor talk about "morphine," it reminded me of my mother, because they prescribed it when her cancer advanced. They also wanted to put her in hospice, but I wouldn't hear of it.

"She's coming home with me," I told the doctor. "I can set her up in my living room and hire a private nurse. In the night I'll give her the morphine shots myself."

"But don't you run a day care downstairs in your home?" he said.

"Yes, but I can still take care of it."

And by the grace of God, I had. One night, however, after I gave Mom her morphine shots, she started hollering, "Get the cookies out of the oven. Grandma's coming for dinner!"

I dabbed her forehead. "No, Mom. Grandma's with Jesus. Remember, we said our good-byes at her funeral when I was ten."

A couple days later, Mom looked at the wedding photos of her and Daddy and saw something else. Something fearful. "Take them down!" she ordered. Of course, I'd do anything to calm her. But oh, how I hated those morphine shots. Hated them for the hallucinations they gave.

I tried to soothe Mom by singing songs we used to sing with my sisters when we baked bread and cookies together. When those didn't help, I played old cassette tapes of us singing at family reunions. What I wouldn't do to pull her back to a place of peace and warmth.

"Mom, do you feel my arms around you? That's Jesus and me hanging on to you." And that's how she slipped into his arms — with Jesus and me at her side.

Three days later, I had to cover Mom's empty bed so I could host Jason's long-awaited high school graduation party. We didn't have time to dispose of her bed before the big celebration, so there it sat — smack in the middle of our living room — an unplanned reminder of how God offered fresh possibilities in the midst of gut-wrenching lows.

And now, as Dr. Noll wrote out a prescription for morphine, I saturated my pain with prayer:

In every passing moment, God, you have a future plan. Thank you for showing me how to pray even as I return to this medicine. And please protect me from having hallucinations.

Dr. Noll sent me to a new physical therapist to work on my hands.

"Physical therapy never worked on my foot," I told her.

"I know," she said, "but this time we're working in a different area."

I closed my eyes as the needle pierced my neck for the pain block.

"You'd better wait a few minutes," I said. "In case the numbing doesn't last."

She smiled reassuringly. "I'm sure it will be just fine."

"No, really," I pressed. "Pain blocks wear off really fast with me."

She talked to me to calm me, but she still went back to work, stretching and manipulating my already swollen fingers. Three minutes later, I gritted my teeth. "I feel it!"

How many tears did I have left in my cocoon of endless pain?

·—※—·

Weary of traditional medicine, I decided to spread my wings and fly in a different direction by going to see a chiropractor. Dr. Dale Chambers used the ol' hands-on crack-and-crunch technique.

"I'll be as gentle as possible," he said. But he knew RSD only from a textbook.

After several visits and adjustments, he gave me a regretful look. "This isn't working. Your body has a mind of its own. Whenever I adjust you, your spine goes right back to the same position."

"So that's it then?"

He nodded. "I'm sorry I wasn't able to help you."

I sighed. "It's not your fault. It's nobody's fault. It's this stubborn ol' body. Man, I can't wait for that day when I'll get a new one." Realizing what that might sound like, I assured him, "Don't worry—I always take one day at a time. God's in control."

He wore a slight frown. "You make it hard for me to tell you what I need to say next."

"Go ahead," I told him.

"Well, I hate to say this, but if Dr. Noll doesn't put your hip and back in a brace, I'm afraid you're going to lose them."

My voice cracked. "Lose my back and hip? How? I mean ... I can't imagine ..."

He curled his lips under. "Of course you can't—and you shouldn't. That's why I mailed Dr. Noll a letter telling him the same thing I'm telling you: He needs to get you in a brace as soon as possible. You're already starting to shift." With that, he blew out a long, tired breath. "All I can say is, I hope he takes my warning seriously."

Bitter Cup

November 1995

When Dr. Noll stepped in for my appointment, he held Dr. Chambers' letter in his hand. "Do you know about this?"

"Know about it?" I said. "I've hardly been able to stop thinking about it."

"Well, I don't want you to worry," he said. "I've been working with you a lot longer than this chiropractor, and I don't think it's time to give you a hip and back brace."

"You don't?"

"No, I don't. You do need something else, though." He shifted on his feet. "I've been watching the changes in your left hand, and we definitely need to do something about those crutches. They're ruining your hands and shoulders."

My voice cracked. "Do something? Like what?"

"Well, for starters, we're going to prescribe some special attachments. They're horizontal armrests that connect to your crutches. What you do is, you strap in your forearms with Velcro and then the tape holds them in there."

"Sounds lovely," I said flatly.

He held his gaze. "We don't want you to keep putting all that pressure on your hands and fingers. Frankly, it looks like they're already trying to claw. I'd hate to see you lose your hand from all that constant pressure."

My mouth went dry. First my back and hip—and now my hand? "Of course I'll use them," I said. "Maybe they're just what I need. Maybe they'll help."

※

A few weeks later, while Ellie pulled out my boxes of garlands, lights, and nativities, I struggled with my crutches. "Can you please do up my Velcro?" I asked. She was used to me making a lot of requests, but fastening crutch attachments was a new one. Frankly, I'd never seen anybody use them before. And they looked as ridiculous as they felt.

After I moved my forearm in place, she strapped it in. "Thanks," I said. I took a few mechanical clumsy steps and paused to rest. "Man, it hurts to use these things."

"I'm sorry," she said, straightening an angel's dress. "I hope it works out. Do you want all your angels on the risers this year?"

"Absolutely."

So one by one, we pulled them out of their boxes and set them on the wooden stand Ellie's husband had made. It felt good to make progress. Lo and behold, my apartment was beginning to look a lot like Christmas.

※

On Christmas Eve, Jeff, Jason, Tara, and I gathered around my table to celebrate.

"Let's pray," I said. *"Father, we thank you for another year where we can celebrate your goodness and grace. Thanks for this sweet baby boy or girl that's growing in Tara's womb. Please keep Tara healthy and strong, and the baby too. May everything go smoothly for all the rest of her pregnancy and delivery. And thank you for this delicious food we're about to enjoy. In Jesus' name. Amen."*

As we dug into the ham, potatoes, salads, and fresh-out-of-the-oven dinner rolls, we joked and chatted about my favorite topic in the world: babies, of course. Tara's voice picked up when she talked about holding her firstborn for the first time.

"How exciting to focus on a baby at Christmas," I said.

Tara nodded. "Please pass the rolls, Uncle Jeff."

"Sure, but let me pass them to Grandma first." And he gave me a wink.

The word "Grandma" warmed me all over, but it also came with the shooting arrow of fear. What if my hand became permanently clawed like the doctor talked about? Would I even be able to hold my new little grandbaby? Worse yet—what if the chiropractor was right about my back becoming permanently bent and crooked? The very thought knotted my stomach. How would I be able to play in the park and do all the fun things I'd dreamed of?

Stop it, I told myself. That'll never happen. You'll be just fine.

Well, maybe I would, maybe I wouldn't, but by the time the four of us moved into the living room, my stomach was anything but fine. It was doing somersaults, flip-flops, and cartwheels all at the same time.

Father, what have I done? Have I worried myself sick?

I slowly breathed in and out as Jason and Jeff handed out presents from under the tree.

Tara peeled off the wrapping. "Ooo ... look. It's a Mickey Mouse doll. Thanks, Uncle Jeff."

I tried to sound jovial. "Oh, sweet. I'm sure the baby will love him." I didn't breathe a word about how horrible I felt. I didn't want to spoil the fun for others. Besides, nobody else seemed to have this strange stomach sickness.

What's going on, God? You feel this with me, don't you? Nobody else knows about it, but I'm glad I can talk to you. I don't know about my Christmas meal, God. It was delicious, but I think I'm beginning to regret it ...

Restricted

January 1996

"I think it's the drugs," the gastrointestinal specialist said. "They've done a number on your stomach."

I rubbed my hand near my neck. "Are we talking permanent damage?"

He nodded. "I believe so."

"Okay," I said, trying to swallow, "what do you suggest?"

"Protein drinks. These days they come in all different flavors, so you have a lot to choose from."

I didn't care if they came in banana split and Oreo cookie. Nothing about them sounded in the least bit appetizing, and I sure couldn't imagine taking them in the place of regular meals. Goodness, I'd always had a big hearty appetite to keep up with my active lifestyle. I still needed a lot of energy—except for different reasons. Now I needed it to get from one doctor to the next.

Choose thankfulness, the Lord reminded me in a whisper. And that helped me remember Psalm 28:7, a psalm I'd been returning to a lot lately: "The LORD is my strength and my shield; my heart trusts in him, and he helps me. My heart leaps for joy, and with my song I praise him."

Okay, God, I choose to sing your praise.

✳

As the days began to feel longer, however, the songs competed with my pain. One afternoon, as I struggled to get comfortable, Daddy left the bedroom and came back with a plain wooden board about two and a half feet long.

I laughed. "What's that for?"

"I'm not exactly sure yet," he said, "but I think we might be able to relieve your pain if we use this to adjust your position."

Leave it to Daddy to come up with a unique idea. Ellie set the board on the bed. "Let's see if it gives you any extra support." We placed it near the headboard and they helped me sit on it — but the bed simply had too much flexibility and movement for the board to do anything.

Daddy then wedged the board flat across the windowsill, away from the glass. "Look, it fits perfectly right in here. Well, you can at least give it a try," he said, ignoring my raised eyebrow.

I hurt too much to argue, so I let the two of them help me plant my bottom on the old rugged slab, my back to the glass. It took a few tries, but after balancing myself just right, the thing actually gave me some relief.

"Praise the Lord!" Daddy said.

"Amen," I agreed. "What a beautiful ugly plank." And I felt so much relief that tears poured down my cheeks.

At my next appointment, I looked up at Dr. Noll as he clasped his hands under his chin. "Ema, the crutch attachments aren't working like we hoped. I think we need to be done with these."

"But I've only used them for a few weeks."

"I know, but that should be more than enough time to see if they're working."

I drew in a breath. "So what do we do now?"

"That's what I want to talk to you about," he said.

My heart beat fast whenever I stood at a new crossroad. "Go on."

"With the pain spreading to your hands, arms, and shoulders, I think it's time for a change. I think we need to switch you to Dr. Keith Bengston in the upper-extremity department. Once the pain climbs above your waist, it's a whole new ball game. Don't worry, though. Dr. Bengston is an expert, and he's very knowledgeable about RSD."

✳

Dr. Noll was right about Dr. Bengston knowing what he was talking about. His voice sounded calm and gentle, and his eyes twinkled when he smiled. I liked him instantly. As he adjusted his glasses, he ran a hand over his balding head and invited me to tell him about the pain.

"Oh, boy," I said. "Would you like me to start with my head and work my way down?"

He sniffed a laugh. "However you like."

When I told him about my hands, he wanted me to soak them in warm water. "It will relax them during therapy," he said. "It will also show us how they respond."

Oh, I knew how they responded all right. Contact with water, wind, and clothing could cause any degree of burning, shooting pain. As much as I hated to admit it, even hugs hurt. As a natural-born hugger, I doubted I'd ever let that stop me though.

Dr. Bengston set a large white bucket on the table in front of me. "This will take about fifteen minutes."

"Okay." I gritted my teeth like a child being forced to smile for a photo. If I wanted to survive this, I'd have to focus on something pleasant to distract myself from the pain. So as I dipped my hands in the water bucket, I thought back to my day care days—back to a time when God used another type of bucket to bail me out.

When Susie's mother dropped her off for day care the first time, she gave me a warning: "Susie throws up. Not just a little, but all the time."

I'd dealt with a lot of behavioral issues over the years, but never

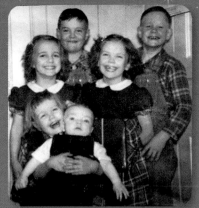

Here I am, surrounded by siblings,
holding my brother Murray.

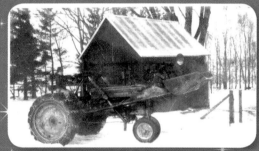

This is the woodshed where my
sister, Mary Lois, and I were
burned when a stove toppled over.

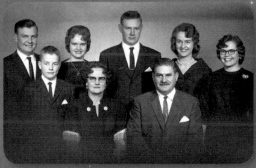

The McKinley family.

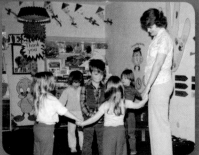

Loving every minute with
my day care children.

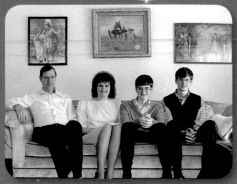

Eddie, me, Jeff, and Jason Lano.

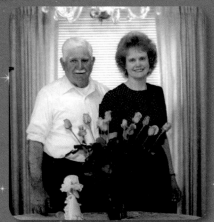

Cherishing my beloved Daddy.

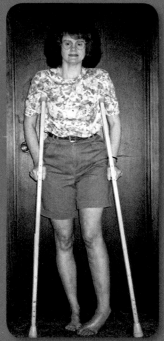

Shortly after the 1993
accident that changed
my life forever.

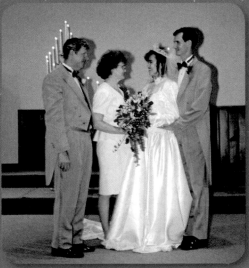

Hobbling around at my son Jason's wedding.

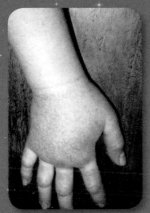

My hands often became puffy and swollen.

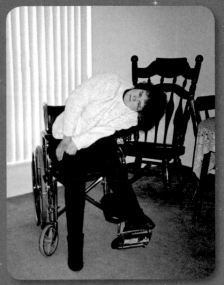

Sadly, nothing could stop my spine from curving to the side.

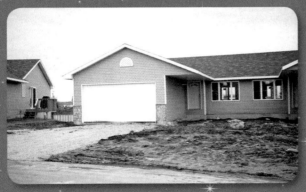

My townhome while under construction.

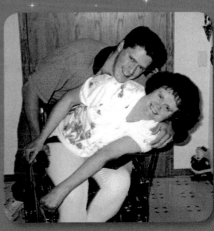

Posing with Bill Butts, my R&S Transport driver.

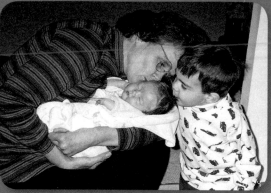

Enjoying my grandsons—Brady and
his baby brother Connor.

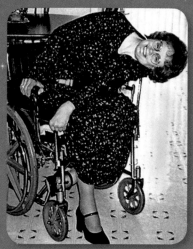

I always tried my best to smile.

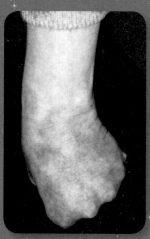

Eventually I couldn't move the
fingers on my left hand, and it
closed in a permanent fist.

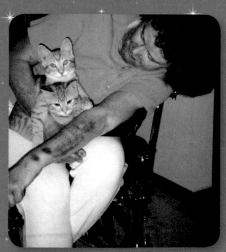

God gave me a sweet gift
in Max and Savannah.

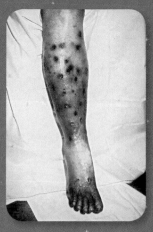

Due to infections, blood clots, and darkened toes, doctors urged amputation of my right leg to save my life. I refused.

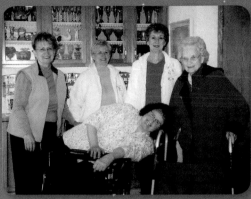

Hanging around with my cousins Joyce, Daisy, Jane, and my Aunt Grace.

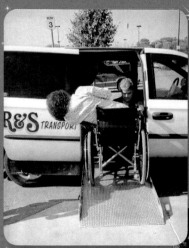

My extreme tilt made it tough to fit through the door of the R&S van.

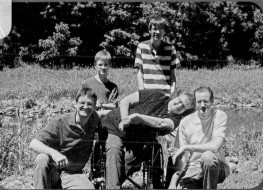

Capturing memories with my sons Jeff and Jason, and my grandsons Connor and Brady.

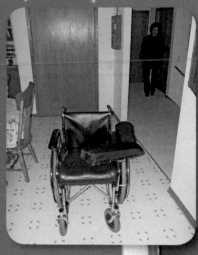

"Isn't that Grandma's wheelchair?"
exclaimed grandson Connor.

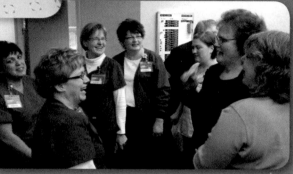

Nurses clamored to see my miracle firsthand.

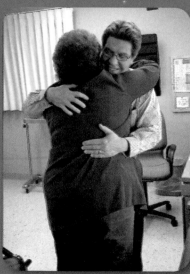

The big moment when I revealed
my new self to my primary
doctor, Dr. David Bell.

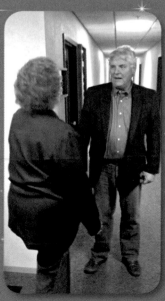

I surprised my attorney, Charlie Bird,
when I actually "walked" into his office.

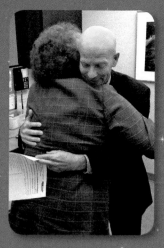

Dr. Keith Bengston, my longtime RSD doctor, wrapped me in a gentle hug when he saw my miraculous transformation.

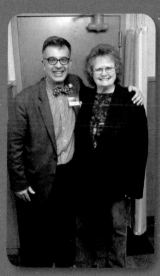

Gastroenterologist, Dr. Amindra Arora, recovered from shock to pose for a photo.

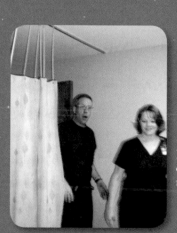

Dermatologist, Dr. Clark Otley, couldn't believe it when he saw me standing there healed.

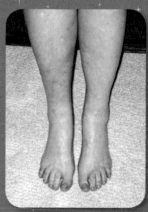

Healed—the left foot is as straight as the right foot.

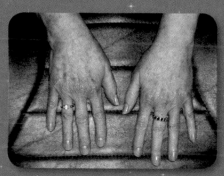

Healed—new skin covers raw areas, no more club left hand.

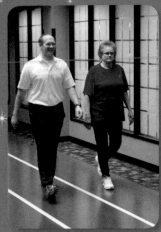

I can now walk the track with my trainer.

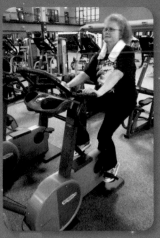

I can work out at the gym.

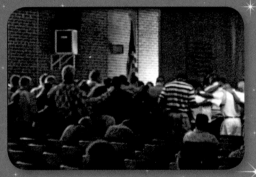

I can give talks like this one at the Salvation Army Rehabilitation Center where men struggling with addiction came forward for prayer.

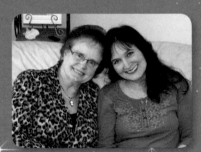

I'm thankful for *Rush of Heaven* writer Cheryl Ricker.

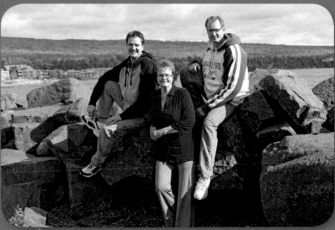

I love standing with sons Jeff and Jason— living proof of God's awesome miracle.

that one. And unfortunately, Susie's mother was right. The four-year-old threw up so much that I could have easily spent the whole day on a big cleanup mission. But thankfully, God gave me good ideas as easily as prayers.

I got down on Susie's level to tell her a secret. "Susie, I'm going to give you a very special ice-cream bucket. It's all yours. And look, it's even got your name on it. From now on, whenever you want to throw up, that's fine with me. Just make sure you always use your very special ice-cream bucket."

Susie looked from me to the bucket, then grabbed it and ran off. Following her, I hid behind the corner to watch. She gingerly fingered the handle, taking ownership of her bucket. And thank the dear Savior of the universe: Susie liked her new ice-cream bucket too much to mess with it. In other words, right then and there, she dropped her old throw-up habit.

"It's not fair," her mother said. "I spent six weeks in intensive therapy trying to deal with this — and you solved it with an ice-cream bucket?"

I shrugged. "I asked God for wisdom and he gave it to me."

I sighed as Dr. Bengston manipulated my hands in the water. If only God would give one of us a better idea right now. One that definitely didn't involve a water bucket.

After we finished, my hands looked puffier than before we started. I felt like Susie's mom when she said, "No fair," except I pressed myself to say something else:

Yes, you are fair, my Father. "Surely, LORD, you bless the righteous; you surround them with your favor as with a shield" (Psalm 5:12).

―✳―

On my next visit with Dr. Bengston, he drew in his lips. "I'm very sorry," he said. "In addition to having RSD in your feet, legs, hands, arms, and shoulders, I think you also have it in your neck and spine."

My hands balled into fists. Wasn't that what the chiropractor had said when he tried to warn Dr. Noll? He even sent him a letter. And I too had tried to warn him about this. I didn't think Dr. Bengston could say anything worse, but I was wrong.

"We do need to get you off your crutches, though," he said. "See the way you're hanging off them? They're ruining your back, neck, and shoulders."

"But Dr. Noll gave them to me. He even tried attachments. What else could we do?"

He took a long breath and blew it out slowly. "That's what I have to talk to you about, Ema. Your widespread RSD is affecting your whole skeletal structure. I think it's time to move you into a wheelchair."

I froze. Everything in me wanted to cry out in protest. Oh, how I wished I hadn't heard him correctly, but I knew I had. A wheelchair? I felt sentenced for a crime I didn't commit.

God, where are you? I've been praying for healing, but we're moving in the wrong direction. I've always been the strong independent one. Remember me—the one who loves to help others in their wheelchairs? Not the other way around.

I cleared my throat. "Are you sure?"

Dr. Bengston nodded.

Of course he was sure. Why else would he have said it? Besides, if I took an honest look at my body, didn't the pain speak for itself? Even now, it felt like an invisible weight wanted to pull me over.

He searched my eyes. "How are you doing?"

"I don't know," I said. "But can I ask you a question?"

"Sure. Anything. Go ahead."

"How did my RSD get so out of control? I mean, why couldn't we have stopped it from traveling?"

He thought for a second. "Well, we don't really know, but it's possible that the intensity of therapy kept your pain in a vicious cycle and made it more difficult for your body to get better."

His answer felt like a punch, and I wanted to scream, *Why did they do it then?* But I already knew the answer. They did it because they didn't know what else to do. When it came to RSD, the doctors really had only two choices: medication and therapy. Since every case was so unique, I ended up being their guinea pig.

"God will help me get through this," I said.

Even as the words fell out of my mouth, I wondered how exactly he would.

Caregivers

February 1996

Old stores and buildings blurred by as Daddy drove downtown to get my wheelchair. The thought of losing my mobility hounded me like a cry in the night. How had it come to this? And why hadn't God reversed things?

"Lord, give us strength," Daddy prayed.

As he pulled into the parking lot, it struck me: how would I leave the store? On crutches or in my new wheelchair? The crutches caused constant pain, but the wheelchair? Well, I could hardly stand to think of it.

The door squeaked open to every brand, shape, and size of wheelchair you could imagine lining the store walls from top to bottom.

"Maybe you can help me," I said, handing the man my prescription.

"Looks like you need a sixteen-incher. No problem." He grabbed a ladder and shot up the steps. "Here she is. Let's give this baby a whirl."

Daddy took my crutches while the guy got it down and wheeled it behind me.

I painfully lowered myself to the seat. "I don't know about this," I said.

"How's it feel, ma'am?"

I shrugged. "Horrible and great."

He nodded. "It takes time to get used to, but don't worry. We can always make adjustments."

Daddy set his hand on my shoulder. "Shall I push you to the car?"

So that was that. Three incredibly long years after my accident, I was now confined to a wheelchair.

With loss of my mobility came the need for full-time caregivers. After getting in touch with an agency, they sent me Sue, Shannon, Hazel, Lisa, Kristen, and Tammy. They dropped in one at a time, like gifts that kept coming and going. And boy, did I have fun trying to keep up with their names and schedules. Some of them worked six or seven hours at a stretch; others, two or three. Either way, my apartment never stopped buzzing with questions and instructions while we all adjusted to my new normal.

Lord, I feel like my space has been invaded. If possible, can we narrow it down to just a couple workers with long, steady hours?

Tammy was the first caregiver to take me shopping. She joined me in the R&S Transport van for a fun jaunt to Shopko. While she touched up her makeup, I joked with Bill Butts, the kind young driver. We got so into our conversation that I couldn't believe how fast the time flew before we pulled into the parking lot. "Now don't go and buy the store out," he quipped.

"Ha, I'll try my best."

As Tammy wheeled me inside the store, I felt strange shopping with somebody other than Ellie. But like everything else, I'd get used to it.

"I'd like us to start in the kitchen department," I said. "Then we can work our way to cleaning goods."

She nodded. But after taking me to the pots and pans, she quickly excused herself. "I'll be right back."

She left so fast I assumed she needed to use the restroom. No problem. I could handle that. Besides, I was used to waiting.

While I watched people pick up their items and examine them, I remembered my Garretts days, back when I used to climb ladders and carry a squirt gun. The good ol' days.

I looked at my watch. Ten minutes had come and gone. Hopefully, she wasn't in trouble. I couldn't imagine pulling her out of a stall or something.

As my aisle grew busier, people had to walk around me. I tried moving out of the way, but as soon as I did, I ended up blocking someone else. Clearly, I needed more practice at this wheelchair thing.

Fifteen minutes passed. Where was she? People started looking irritated, and I didn't blame them. An older woman waved her hand. "Can I help you, dear?"

Absolutely, I wanted to say. You can either take me home or make an announcement: *Missing caregiver to the front desk, please.* Instead, I looked at the woman and smiled. "No, thank you. I'm sure my friend will be back in a minute."

And yes, she was—with four big shopping bags in her arms!

"Oh, my gosh," she said, sounding winded. "The sales are just ridiculous."

It felt like someone had turned up the heat. "Tammy, I can't believe you just did that. The agency isn't paying you to shop. What did you think I'd do, just sit around and enjoy myself? It's not like I can push a shopping cart from my wheelchair."

She looked shocked that I'd actually call her on it, but what did she expect—that I'd get excited about her purchases? Great, I thought. Now I might have to report her. I didn't want to get anybody in trouble, but I also didn't want this to happen to others.

Oh, Father, I'm sorry. I just lost it with Tammy. Please shine your grace and goodness on all this. In spite of me.

——✳——

Two weeks later, I noticed that my new bottle of morphine pills was half empty. My heart sank. Had I taken too many? Or worse: was I losing my mind?

Father, I don't know what to do or what's going on. Please show me.

A couple hours later, the agency called. "By any chance, have your medications been going down extra fast?"

I squeezed the phone tightly. "What do you mean?"

"I'll be blunt," she said. "We have good reason to believe that one of our caregivers has been stealing people's drugs."

"Oh, thank goodness!"

"Excuse me?"

I laughed. "No, it's just that mine have been going down extra fast and I'm rather relieved my brain isn't."

"Anyway," she said, indignantly, "Hazel won't be coming back. You'll be getting a replacement."

The agency sent me a young mother named Cathy Ruggeberg. And oh, what a blessing! From the moment Cathy walked in with her bouncy red hair and servant-like attitude, I could tell she wanted to give it only her best. She and Ellie hit it off like sisters, which pleased me too. I could hardly wait to offer Cathy more hours.

Thank you, Jesus, for taking such good care of me.

Still, I dreamed of a day when I wouldn't need caregivers anymore. A day when I'd be so normal that I could be a caregiver myself. Maybe even start my own agency.

Leaning

June 1996

"Grandma's empty arms are waiting . . ."

As Jason stood up from the couch, he glanced at Tara, then parked in front of my wheelchair.

"Here you go." He tucked little Brady in my arms, and I took a deep breath of his baby smells. My eyes welled as I drank in the sight of him. I couldn't have been more smitten by this two-month-old little love bundle. "You're perfect," I told him.

I had imagined these moments differently. Clearly, I had never imagined I'd be holding my first grandchild with my left hand completely closed in a fist. A club hand, they called it.

My upper body now leaned into what Cathy called a half-moon. My left shoulder rested in a trough-like attachment and my neck cocked to the side on a lopsided tilt.

But thank you, Jesus, that I can still use my good hand to caress his dark little tussle of hair.

"He's sleepy," I said, watching his eyes open and close. It would have been nice to pace the floor with him, maybe even give him a bounce or two, but at least I could bounce him on the inside. I wouldn't let anything spoil our time together. Not even if Brady messed his diaper or fussed. I was too much in love.

I sang without reservation: "Jesus loves the little children, all the children of the world. Red and yellow, black, and white, they are precious in his sight. Jesus loves the little children of the world."

Jason looked amused. "What are you going to do next—read to him?"

I puffed my lips. "Hmm, good idea. Give me a book."

He knew I'd do it too, but we'd have time for that later.

As I held Brady awkwardly, his body nestled against mine as if it was meant to be there. "This is what you call grandma therapy," I said. "And just look at him. Look how he leans into me with such perfect trust. He's the total picture of peace."

✳

The following week brought more pain, and I needed to lean into Jesus like Brady leaned into me—especially when I saw Dr. Bengston and he explained that I was leaning more in a literal sense.

"We need to make a few wheelchair adjustments," he said. "For starters, I think we need to adjust your armrest. And since your right hip doesn't quite hit the chair and your left foot always wants to tuck under, I think we also need to move your footrest. And maybe lower your shoulder piece as well."

Boy, did I ever sound like a mess. Suddenly, I felt quite sorry for the man. "How do you do it?" I asked. "How do you hold it together when you see people like me deteriorate so quickly? I mean, doesn't it break your heart?"

He smiled. "Yes, but this is what I do. I can't let myself focus on how fast people go down. I need to save my energy to help them get better."

"So that's your secret then? Focus?"

He shrugged. "What I want to know is, what's *your* secret? How do you always stay so positive?"

I laughed. "I keep leaning on Jesus. I figure if he could die on the cross for me two thousand years ago, the least I can do is give him the gift of my heart. And that includes my heart's attitude of trust—which, believe me, I'm still working on each and every day."

That same day, I had to see Dr. Clause, my primary doctor. I arrived extra early so I could take it easy, relax, and maybe even pray. It always took a lot of courage to see all these doctors because, frankly, you never knew what was going to happen next.

A little boy in the waiting room inched closer on the couch to check me out. Our eyes met, and I melted into his bright little pools of blue.

He pointed at my club hand on the armrest. "What happened?"

"Andrew James!" his mother yelled. "Get back here!"

I gasped. "Oh, please don't. He's fine. Oh, my goodness, I'd stare at me too if I was him."

Completely ignoring me, she yanked his arm and talked sharply in his ear. Man, I hated it when parents did that. I tried to wave and get her attention. "Excuse me. Ma'am? It doesn't bother me. Not at all. I'm just happy to connect." But she'd already stuck her nose back in her magazine.

An older woman on the couch, however, responded to my wish to connect. "I have fibromyalgia," she said. "The pain's invisible, but real."

I instantly wanted to hug her. "I'm sorry," I said. "I've heard it's awfully painful." I considered telling her about my RSD, but decided against it because how would that really help her? Besides, what would I say? *Hi, I have RSD. It's the most painful of all neurological disorders. Matter of fact, it sits right up there on the top of the pain pyramid. Oh, and it has the highest suicide rate.* True as this was, what would that accomplish—other than to maybe trivialize her pain?

I did my best to listen and give her my full attention. And the more I did, the more I found my own screaming pain quiet down.

"See these bags?" she said, pointing under her eyes. "I have a hard time sleeping at night."

"I know the feeling," I said. "Would you mind if I prayed for you?"

Her eyes widened. For a second I thought she'd say no, but instead she said, "Sure. Why not."

"Remind me your name?" I said.

"It's Melanie."

"Okay, let's pray, Melanie. *Father, I thank you for my new friend, Melanie. I ask that you heal her body, take away her pain, and help her to be able to sleep. Also, please give her and her doctor peace and wisdom during this appointment. In Jesus' name. Amen.*"

When I looked up, she dabbed her eyes with a Kleenex. "Thanks for the prayer. Nobody's ever done that for me before."

"Well, you deserve to feel special. God loves you very much."

It felt good to help someone. Lately, however, I'd been feeling something brooding in my own heart. Something dark that I really didn't want to touch.

Lord? Do I need a little extra help, myself?

Forgiveness

July 1996

As Cathy, my caregiver, backed out of Dr. Dave Stensland's office to give us privacy, I stole a glance at his psychology diplomas on the wall.

Yes, I reminded myself, it makes sense to take Dr. Clause's advice and come here for help.

It was bound to happen anyway. Because of the severe physical pain associated with RSD, they expected primary-care doctors to refer us to psychologists.

"Great to meet you, Ema." Dr. Dave's warmth instantly relaxed me. He looked trustworthy, but I especially liked seeing the well-worn Bible on his desk.

He leaned back in his chair. "I'd love to hear a little bit about Ema," he said.

"Sure. Well, first I'll tell you—I love Jesus. He and I have been together for a really long time."

"Great," he said. "I can relate to that. How long have you been a Christian?"

"Since I was seventeen, a senior in high school."

He looked pleased. "Such a key time in a young girl's life. Would you like to talk about it?"

His words gave me all the permission I needed to let the memories spill. I told him about the house on the hill and how it all started with Daddy telling us, "We're going to Grandpa's church tonight."

I wasn't happy about it. "On a school night?" I said. "I have a mountain of homework and my hair's frizz city."

But Daddy wouldn't be moved. "It's a special service, and Grandpa invited us to join him."

The way I looked at it, we already attended church once a week. We didn't need to supplement it. I loved the people in our little country church. We were like family. Once, when I was ten, a tornado hit on a Sunday morning. Part of our building crumbled while my Sunday school class huddled under a big table in the church basement. There, we recited Bible verses like our lives depended on it. That was cool and everything, but I didn't need to visit another church, especially on a school night.

"I don't want to go," I told them plainly.

"Well, I'm sorry," Mom said, "but it's not up for negotiation. We're going as a family." And that was that.

So I sat in the back with my arms crossed, staring at the clock.

The preacher preached so loud and fiery that I couldn't have fallen asleep if I'd wanted to. "Hell is a place God designed for Satan and his demons. It's a place of eternal fear and torment. A place where the fire never goes out ..."

I shuddered. And here I thought sitting in church was bad.

"Heaven, on the other hand," he said, "is a place of love, peace, and joy—the kind you experience when you start your relationship with Jesus."

He talked about Jesus like he and the big guy were best buds, which really got me thinking: Did I really know God like that, or did I just know *about* him?

The more this dude spoke, the more something stirred. That's probably why I nearly froze when he looked in my direction to make his next point.

"If you're feeling something stirring inside you—that's the Holy Spirit. He's working on your heart, drawing you closer to Jesus."

If I was stirred before, now I could hardly sit. My eyes stayed on the preacher as he made eye contact around the room. "If you'd like a relationship with Jesus, please step out of your seats and join us at the front."

"I love it," Dr. Dave said. "Did you go forward?"

"I was one of the first people down the aisle, and Jesus and I have been best friends ever since."

Dr. Dave smiled. "Wonderful. And did that decision change your life?"

"Oh, yeah ... I couldn't wait to tell my friends about my new commitment. And they could tell right away that something had happened. I began to take my faith very seriously."

He pointed at my wheelchair. "Want to talk about this?"

My body stiffened. I'd go there if it helped, but I really didn't want to. I took a long, deep breath and let the night pour out of me: the store, the boxes, the so-called friends.

He shook his head. "It's a miracle you even survived. Has anybody ever told you you're a T.O.B?"

I gave him a funny look. "A what?"

He wrote down the letters: T.O.B.

I laughed. "No, I don't believe anybody's ever called me a T.O.B."

"Well, you're a tough old bird, that's what you are."

"Hmm, I kinda like that. Does that mean we're finished — now that I know what I am?"

He grinned. "In God's timing. First, I'd like to ask you something, and this question is a bit more serious."

"Go for it," I said.

"Okay. How did you manage to forgive all those people who let you down that night? All those people who forgot about you?"

I shrugged. "I don't know. I just did it, I guess."

He rubbed his chin. "Well, if you're okay with it, I'd like you to do a little exercise that might help us."

"Sure, as long as you don't want me to do a reenactment."

He stayed serious. "I want you to close your eyes and go back to the night of the accident when everything happened. Can you do that for me?"

I nodded. "I can already picture everything as if I'm there."

"Okay, good. Who do you see, Ema? I want you to picture each person who let you down that night."

It didn't take long for me to see their faces. Suddenly the resentment I'd tried to push down so many times since the accident felt like lava—burning and no longer containable. My crooked body began to shake with sobs.

"We're a safe place to let out our emotions." He handed me a Kleenex. "Don't worry. We're going in a good direction, and I think God wants to make room for more forgiveness. With more forgiveness comes more emotional healing, and that's what we all want."

As the words erupted out of me, I sucked in gasps of air. I told him about Lana, who was supposed to drive me home that night. She knew I needed a ride. I'd even verified it. Why did she assume I'd go home on my own without telling her? And what about the other staff who cleaned up the huge mess I'd left on the floor? How could they assume I'd leave the place in such a shamble? That wasn't my way. And Rick, my manager—he was there, but he didn't even check the time clock to see if I'd clocked out. They were all about to leave without knowing what happened to me. These were the people I'd always helped and cared for. And I could have so easily died because of their carelessness.

Before I left, Dr. Dave gave me some homework. He wanted me to write a letter to each of the people who overlooked me that night. They'd never see it, of course, but it would help me get in touch with my hidden emotional pain so I could release each person to God. It would take a little time, yes, but he assured me it would be worth it.

If anybody could heal my heart, God could. Even before the accident, he had a plan to get me through this. Not only that, but Jesus knew exactly what it felt like to be abandoned by friends and left hanging.

When I got home, I spent several hours writing those letters and spilling out my heart to Jesus. After I finished, a feeling of lightness washed over me as I lifted each person to God. And not just those behind my accident at Garretts, but also Tammy, the caregiver who left me stranded in Shopko, my ex-husband, and even Vance Wade.

Lord, forgive them all. And forgive me for not forgiving them.

As the prayers gushed out of me, I no longer felt bound by my resentment at the way these people had treated me. Instead, I felt fresh freedom, the kind that comes only from forgiving others and myself. Relishing this gift, I wondered what the Lord would have me do next.

Purpose

October 1996

As Cathy parked my wheelchair at the back of the church, pulsing music pressed my migraine. "My church days are numbered," I'd warned my pastor in a recent home visit. "Because of my RSD, the lights and music wreak havoc on my stress levels." He'd told me he understood, but how could anybody, really?

Fresh sadness crept over me, because somehow I knew this would be my last day. The hugs had taken a toll. So had the voices pounding in my ears. And oh, man, the lights. With my head cocked to the side, I was a sitting target. It was definitely time to start listening online.

The sounds faded and Pastor Steer took the podium, greeted us in his warm British accent, and plunged into his sermon with passion. My heart quickened when he flashed a picture on the screen: that famous old painting of Jesus knocking on the door.

"Why is there no handle on Jesus' side?" he asked. "Because Jesus gives us the choice about whether or not we want to open to him. In Revelation 3:20 he says, "Here I am! I stand at the door and knock. If anyone hears my voice and opens the door, I will come in . . .""

As he neared the end of his message, I suddenly felt a fresh sensitivity to the people around me. That teenage girl in the red dress — did she know Jesus? That older man with the snow-white hair — would I see him in heaven someday? The more my eyes scanned the crowd, the more God's love welled up inside me. I didn't even have to stir it up. It was just there. I found myself praying for every man, woman, boy, and girl.

Oh, God, don't let any of them leave this place without finding the kind of love, joy, and peace that you've given me.

It had been a long time since I prayed with such desperation, but I knew I wasn't just throwing my thoughts in the air. God heard each one. And like he said in James 5:16, "The prayer of a righteous person is powerful and effective." God heard my prayer. Not because I was righteous — at least not on my own apart from him — but rather because I had a relationship with him. The righteous one clothed me in *his* righteousness. And because of that, he moved heaven and earth on my behalf.

Cathy stepped in front of me. "Ready to go?"

I don't know how the time slipped away so quickly, but it did, and I felt flooded with emotion.

As soon as I got home, I did something I'd never done before. I went right to our church's website and touched each of the pastors' photos on the screen. There was nothing magical about touching them, but it gave me a point of contact for my prayers, a place where I could stretch my faith. And what a blessing that I could still use one hand to do it.

Father, please use Pastor Steer in a powerful way to reach the community. Please bless those pastors who visit homes, hospitals, and handicapped people like me. And even though I'm in such bad shape physically, thank you that I can always make a difference spiritually. It feels good right down to my hurting toes.

When Thanksgiving rolled around, Bill, the R&S driver, loaded me into the van so Cathy could take me to the Salvation Army.

"How long have you been volunteering for them?" he asked.

"I haven't missed a Thanksgiving or Christmas in fifteen years."

He whistled. "Now that's dedication."

"Serving's addicting," I said. "That's why we see so many of the same volunteers year after year."

But tonight I had other things on my mind. Like how people would respond when they saw me. It had been three and a half years since my accident. When they saw me last year at Christmas, I was on crutches. They probably thought I'd be better by now, not worse. The last thing I wanted was to make people uncomfortable.

"So what's it like?" Bill said. "I mean, what kinds of things do you do with this group?"

"Oh, we have lots of fun." I gave him a glimpse of what Thanksgiving and Christmas used to look like before my accident. How I'd run around serving the big turkey dinner, trying to talk to as many people as possible. Many of the guests smelled like body odor, but we never let their smells get between us. Whether they were homeless or rich, we had only one mission: to make them feel like a million bucks.

The memories grew sweeter when I told Bill how we decorated the tables with beautiful centerpieces. More than one hundred and fifty kids and adults gathered around those tables. Children volunteers made homemade cards and left them at each place setting. And boy, did the kids light up when the guests opened their cards. As we pampered people to the max, I always tried to keep an eagle eye on everything. And when I finally plunked myself down at the table, I made hearty conversation while we dug into our plates with bottomless appetites. It was like a family reunion. And afterward, I served the staff. "You need to feel special too," I told them.

In addition to Christmas meals, we volunteers used to hop in vans and visit the poor. We'd clap our hands, belt out carols, and show up on people's doorsteps with Santa hats on our heads and bells on our toes. We'd stay as long as they let us, which usually turned out to be a long time because they mostly weren't used to getting visitors. We'd give them secondhand clothing, calendars, and fruit baskets. Many were bare-bones poor. They had scraps for furniture and chilly homes, but boy, did those children warm up when we brought them Christmas.

A streak of sadness hit me as I talked about the good ol' days. The days when I could serve food with my own hands. The days when I could jump in and out of a van and even run up people's steps.

"Thanks for sharing," Bill said, bringing the van to a stop. "We need to pull down the ramp. It's time for you to be a blessing again."

Sure enough, when Cathy took me inside, a few volunteers did double takes.

"Ready to go to your post?" Cathy asked.

"You betcha." I was determined to have a good time.

When she wheeled me to the door to greet the guests, a younger couple slipped in with long faces. "Happy Thanksgiving," I said. "I'm glad you could come."

"Happy Thanksgiving to you too," they said, smiling.

A young guy in a hoodie turned up his lip as I greeted him. "What's happy about it? I lost my job and we're barely scraping by."

"Oh, that's hard," I said, nodding with understanding. "I'm very sorry to hear that. But it will turn around and get better—you just wait. In the meantime, there's always something to be thankful for. You hang in there, okay?"

He looked at a loss as he watched me leaning over awkwardly in my wheelchair with a bright smile on my face. He probably thought, *What's* with *this woman anyway?*

He gave me a quick nod and said, "Thanks."

Tom, a regular guest, jumped off his scooter and spread open his arms. "Where's my big squeeze?"

In return, I gave him a lopsided hug. "I'll take it from any angle," I said.

When Major Frye and his wife turned in my direction, their eyes looked sad to see my decline. When I smiled and waved at them, however, they perked up.

"There's our inspirational Ema."

"Ah, you guys are the inspiring ones." And I meant it. Year after year they poured themselves out to serve others. They fully lived out Jesus' words: "It is more blessed to give than to receive."

I didn't want anything more than to live out those words—as long as I could handle it, anyway.

The Fight

December 1996

A few weeks before Christmas, the insurance company gave me an early Christmas surprise: they stopped paying the bills. Whether I liked it or not, Charlie had to fight back. So a judge drove down from the Twin Cities to meet with us in the City Hall conference room in Rochester. This whole court thing had me on edge.

I held my breath as Rick Vanderlin, the lawyer from the other side, stepped into the entryway. The insurance adjuster, Claire Rhodes, pretended she didn't even see me as she passed. Charlie had warned me about her. "You gotta watch that Claire Rhodes. She fights below the belt."

The two of them walked through the open conference room door, while Elizabeth Edwards, the judge, kept an even pace behind them. When she saw me, she stopped. "Here, let me get that second door for you."

I smiled as she opened it. "Thanks."

Cathy pushed me to a long rectangular table beside Charlie. I couldn't help but remember the hot seat. At least this time I had my own little support team.

Daddy, my cousin Daisy, and her husband sat on a bench by the wall. Daddy looked all fired up and ready to go. At least one of us was.

Charlie, Ellie, Cathy, and I sat on one side, while the opposing lawyer, insurance adjuster, and a transcriptionist sat on the other. Judge Edwards took the seat at the end.

Charlie smoothed his suit and straightened his tie before lowering himself behind his tidy stack of papers. Rick Vanderlin didn't look like he'd even combed his hair, and his papers looked all disorganized.

I'd prayed long and hard for this day, but when it came right down to it, God was the ultimate judge.

The last time I met with Charlie, he assured me he'd collected all the right information and hospital documentation. He showed nothing but confidence. But even so, the judge's decision could go either way. If we lost, only God knew what would happen. He'd have to find another way to take care of me.

After a bunch of bantering back and forth, Charlie appealed to the judge. "Your Honor, I'd like to invite you to take a closer look at my client's hand and foot."

Rick Vanderlin shook his head. "I object. We don't need to play on people's emotions. Let's stick with the facts and move on."

"Overruled," the judge said. "It only makes sense that we see what we're talking about." With that, Cathy pulled back my wheelchair, and Judge Edwards walked over to take a closer look.

The room got quiet as she looked at my hand, all curled, swollen, and fused into a fist. I could only imagine what she thought when she bent low to examine my crooked foot. It looked like it had been broken and ignored. Like no one had bothered to set the bones straight. My sad-looking ankle, with my foot bent inward, looked about as useful as a broken hockey stick.

Standing back up, she nodded to Cathy. "You can push her back now. Thanks."

Charlie straightened. "Your Honor, what you see is one of the many effects of progressive widespread RSD that continues to ravage my client's body. It's now left her permanently disabled. As the medical evidence clearly shows, it's the direct result of a work-related accident that never should have occurred. This is why we want the insurance company to do the only right thing and take rightful responsibility."

Enraged, Claire Rhodes slammed her fist on the table. She slammed with such force that she set off all my reflexes. My left hand, tucked safely back under the table, flew up and hit the underside.

I hollered and the judge gasped. "Claire Rhodes, if you don't get a grip on your anger, I'm going to have to ask you to leave. Is that clear?"

"Yes, your Honor."

A normal hand might have eventually bruised, but mine wasn't a normal hand. It took only minutes before it puffed up like an oven roll, which, of course, only added fuel to Charlie's fire.

The court session lengthened, twisted, and turned like a maze. All the while, I felt bone tired and my knees hurt right along with the rest of me.

Finally, Judge Edwards rose to her feet. "Both parties will be notified about my decision in three weeks."

Three weeks? I'd have to ask Charlie if that was normal. Then again, was anything ever normal in my case?

As Cathy took me to the lobby, I made the mistake of looking at Claire Rhodes. Her scowl made me shiver.

Oh, Lord, bless that woman and help her smile. And please give us a good outcome.

I don't know why, but I had a funny feeling about all this. Something told me that no matter what Judge Edwards decided in this case, the insurance people would try to pull something else.

Home

Questions swirled in my mind as Cathy parked me in Charlie's waiting room. What strange news did he want to tell me this time? A couple weeks ago, he told me the insurance company wanted to relocate me to the Twin Cities — stick me in a special program at the Courage Center. Thank goodness, the Courage Center had enough sense to reject me. They told them, "Sorry, she couldn't possibly do this program. We're an independent living facility, and Ema needs constant care." For once I was grateful for my dependence.

I rested my eyes and thanked God for Charlie, who helped me navigate all these things. So far, he'd won every case involving insurance. Because of his legal brilliance, our first settlement had come through a few months earlier. And Charlie had great ideas too. When he saw how much time Ellie spent helping me, he suggested she sign up with an agency and get paid for what she was already doing. So that's exactly what she did.

Cathy and Ellie were the most dependable caregivers I could have asked for. Truly an answer to prayer. Now, if God would only answer the big one and heal me once and for all.

After recently consulting with Dr. Clause about my increasing pain, Dr. Bengston raised my morphine from 300 milligrams to 400 — a whopping amount that sent me running back to Dr. Bengston with my barf bucket and more questions.

I couldn't keep down my protein drinks, so to counteract the nausea, he gave me Zofran. But the Zofran gave me too much stomach acid. So to counteract the Zofran and heartburn, he gave me Prilosec. Getting it right was always a balancing act. Even though I couldn't eat solid foods, my weight constantly went up and down, depending on my medication and its side effects. Sometimes I looked big and bloated. Other times my clothes hung off me like they'd hung on my mom's clothesline.

"Sorry about the wait," Charlie said, opening his door. "Come in."

Charlie looked grim as Ellie maneuvered me to his desk. "It's getting harder for you to fit through doorways, isn't it?"

"I do best with wider ones," I agreed.

"That's what I thought. How do you manage in your little apartment?"

I laughed. "It isn't easy."

He ran a hand over his face. "I think it's time we start talking housing options."

I gave him a look. "They don't want me at the Courage Center, and nursing homes don't have the right-sized doorways. They're meant for wheelchairs, yes, but not for ones with leaning bodies."

He stayed serious. "I'm thinking more along the lines of getting you a small custom-built townhome. What would you think of that?"

I chuckled. "What would I think of it? I think we ought to throw in a trip to the moon."

"I've been researching this, Ema. Because of your disability, you qualify for government assistance. They should be able to cover about half the cost of a decent townhome."

"Get out. Really?" My mind raced. Now *that* would be a dream.

Charlie played with his pen. "I know a couple good builders. We could set you up with Rod and Wayne and get right down to business."

I wanted to hug him on the spot. "Charlie, you've done it again. You've made my entire year."

Over the next few months, God placed other oases in my desert. In addition to constructing a house for me, he also provided me with my own accessible wheelchair van. I could still use R&S, but Cathy and Ellie could also resort to a second option if needed.

Rod and Wayne put together a large work crew and got right to work on my townhome. Several times a week, either Ellie or Cathy drove me to the site so I could watch my blessing take shape.

Thank you, Lord, for building a place especially for me.

It reminded me of heaven. God worked long and hard, preparing a place for me and me for a place. When it got right down to it, everything else was temporary, including my body.

I often thought about 2 Corinthians 5:1: "We know that if the earthly tent we live in is destroyed, we have a building from God, an eternal house in heaven, not built by human hands."

It warmed me to think about my eternal home. How it was more than just a place. It was also a high position. I was seated with Christ in the heavenly places. I was more than just a body. I had a human spirit. And to top it all off, I always had the Holy Spirit. And as long as I said "yes" to Jesus, nothing could possibly take him away. I was safe and sealed by his Holy Spirit within me.

The more I watched the townhome go up, the more I wanted to peek inside. It didn't seem fair that others could go into their homes and add their input, while I had to stay outside because of the steps.

Rod looked understanding when I shared my feelings. "When you come back tomorrow," he said, "we'll have you a makeshift ramp."

True to his word, when I got there the next day, a long plank stretched from the side garage door to the kitchen.

My heart beat wildly as Cathy wheeled me inside. What had once been a complicated blueprint had now morphed into actual rooms.

I loved the size of the kitchen and how it had a deck off to the left.

My new living room veered to the right, and a wide hallway separated the kitchen and living room. A few feet down the hall, I had a bathroom on the left and a bedroom on the right. Since I hadn't slept in a bed for years, I'd save that room for guests.

The room that excited me most was the one at the end of the hall — my own little office.

September 26, 1998

On move-in day, I felt like a queen in her castle. The permanent ramp in the garage was my drawbridge. When Daddy parked me beneath the archway leading to the living room, I could already see where I wanted things to go. We'd stick my plush blue chair in the corner and hang a couple of my Jesus paintings on the bare beige walls.

I especially liked the painting that depicted Matthew 23:37. Jesus is leaning on his staff, overlooking Jerusalem. That's when he said, "Jerusalem, Jerusalem, you who kill the prophets and stone those sent to you, how often I have longed to gather your children together, as a hen gathers her chicks under her wings, and you were not willing."

A knock on the door broke into my thoughts.

"I'll get it," Daddy said. Curious, Ellie followed him.

"Our first guest?" I asked.

Ellie shook her head. "No, Flowers by Jerry."

Sure enough, Daddy returned with a big potted plant and a grin. "It's from Charlie Bird. Our first housewarming gift."

My heart swelled. "You can set it on the kitchen counter. Thanks, Daddy."

Cathy wheeled me through the wide doorway to investigate the bathroom.

"God is so good," I said. "And you know what? This isn't just my home. It's *God's home*. I'm going to dedicate every single room to him. Let's check out my new office."

All she had to do was back me up, take a few steps more, and there we were.

"Your office doesn't have a door," she said.

I laughed. "It doesn't need one."

From my angle, I scanned the upper part of the room and felt a smile stretch across my lips. I could already envision where I wanted my shelves and dolls.

Growing Pains

February 1999

I loved my new house, but somehow, I just couldn't shake a certain fear: What if I had a fire or emergency at night? It's not that I expected to have one ... but what if I did? They always say you're supposed to know in advance what you'd do. Well, would I be able to get out of the house by myself? There was really only one way to find out.

One night, after my caregivers went home, I wheeled myself through the kitchen door and sat at the top of the ramp in the garage. It would take all my strength, but if I gripped the rail, I might just be able to make it down on my own.

So that's what I did. Using my good hand, I squeezed the rail, and inch by painful inch, I made it down. I'll probably pay for this later, I thought. But sure enough, I did it! I made it down.

Then it hit me: *Oh no! How in the world will I get back up?* Great. I'd completely spaced out about that part. The ramp was too steep for me to do it on my own.

Staring at the garage door, I didn't know whether to laugh or cry or do a bit of both. My small cold garage suddenly felt a whole lot smaller and colder. The truth struck like lightning: I'd be stuck here until morning. Until one of my caregivers found me.

Lord Jesus, please hold me. Please speak to me. Please bring some good out of this brain blip.

In those dark, quiet moments, sure enough, he spoke to me. He showed me I'd been burying some more deep-seated feelings of anger and self-pity. Feelings from recent times when others had ignored and misunderstood me. I had to forgive them for that. Again.

Oh, God, you brought me to the base of this cold garage so I could focus on nothing but you. You wanted me to hear from you. Thank you for loving me enough to rebuke me and change me. Thank you for using my stubbornness to show me your stubborn love. Help me be more understanding about people's lack of understanding. By your strength, I choose to forgive again. In Jesus' name. Oh, and thank you for being in control.

Cathy's jaw dropped the next morning when she opened the garage side door. The words came out slowly. "What are you doing down here?"

"Oh, praying," I said. "Beautiful view, don't you think?"

She sighed. "Let's get you back in the house."

"Yeah, let's," I said. "Then maybe I can give you another teeny example of how God works out all things together for good."

※

I loved having company over, especially Daddy, Jeff, Jason, Tara, and, of course, almost-three-year-old little Brady. My grandson brought me joy upon joy. Even from my crooked position, I treasured that I could read him books as well as teach him letters, colors, and numbers, all to help prepare him for school.

One nippy day around Valentine's Day, Jason stopped over with a slight twinkle in his eye.

"What's with you?" I said. "You look happy enough to burst."

He leaned against the kitchen door that opened to the garage and told me matter-of-factly, "We're having another baby."

I felt my hands clasp together at my chest. "Another grandbaby? Oh, my goodness. When?"

"October fifteenth."

I reached out to grab him. "Oh, honey. We need to celebrate."

Ellie and Cathy took me shopping and I beelined for the baby department. I picked up odds and ends like binkies, bottles, and blankets. I'd buy more after the baby came and we knew the gender.

One afternoon, while leafing through Brady's baby album, I got a phone call from Jason.

"Mom, I ..." He sounded stiff. Almost wooden.

"What's wrong? How did it go?"

He sighed. "We had an ultrasound, and there's something wrong with the baby's bones."

"What do you mean?"

"Well, for one thing, he's missing fingers on one of his hands."

I reached for words. "Oh, Jason. I'm sorry ..." I looked at my club hand. How could my grandbaby be missing fingers? My mind spun back to my own pregnancy with Jason, back to the day when they told me about that awful medication. Everything had turned out normal back then. Maybe this was just a mistake.

"It gets worse."

I tried to swallow. "Worse?"

"Yeah, during the ultrasound, the doctor took measurements. The baby's legs and arms are all different lengths. I forget what the doctor called it, but the baby has some kind of bone anomaly."

I sucked in a breath.

Lord Jesus, help me comfort him.

"It's going to be okay, Jason. I'm here for you."

A few hours later, Tara and Jason sat stiffly in my living room. I grabbed Tara's hand, hoping I'd be a comfort. "You know what I think? I think you guys need to get ready because God's giving you an extra special baby."

Tara looked glazed, like she couldn't process the news. Her hands hovered over her stomach like guardians. She patted and rubbed her tummy, making slow even circles, as if the motions themselves would somehow erase the pain.

This felt surreal. Like a nightmare. Although I knew all about bad news, nothing I could say or do felt remotely close to adequate. That's why I did the only sensible thing I could think of. I silently prayed.

July 1999

The more Tara expanded around the middle, the more I leaned to the side. Dr. Bengston added a new contraption to my wheelchair: a head attachment. It was the strangest device I'd ever seen. It jutted out of my wheelchair from a tall steel rod. The concave attachment looked like a trough, and I felt like a horse as my head leaned into it. I used it everywhere. Unfortunately, it made my headaches worse.

"I'm better off hanging," I told Dr. Bengston, a couple weeks later.

"I'm sorry it didn't work out. We'll take it off then."

I sighed with relief. "Thank you."

The poor guy probably didn't know what to do with me. *I* didn't know what to do with me. Hard as I tried, I couldn't even remember what it felt like to be comfortable. Chronic pain had so wound its way into every fabric of my being. I guess you could say I slept with an invisible enemy—except I wasn't sleeping ... or eating ... or doing anything I used to take for granted.

Satan wanted to steal the joy out of me, but I wouldn't let him. Instead, I worked to stay above the water, to plant myself on Jesus, the Rock, and focus on his love and the beauty around me. My Bible became my bread, my manna. I continued to plunge into God's Word, turn its psalms into regular prayers.

"You, LORD, keep my lamp burning; my God turns my darkness into light. With your help I can advance against a troop; with my God I can scale a wall" (Psalm 18:28–29).

I talked to Dr. Dave at least once or twice week. I don't know how he did it, but he somehow made this bent-over woman feel like a hero.

"It's just me," I said. "I'm in process like everybody else, except my process may be taking a little bit longer."

He shook his head. "Most people who face this kind of pain barely scrape by. But look at you, with that true honest-to-goodness smile on your face."

I thought about that for a second. "My pain definitely forces me to turn to God, the source of my strength." I didn't want to sound sappy, but I had something personal to say. "Dr. Dave, you've done an amazing job strengthening me too. God sure knew what he was doing when he directed me to you."

He listened as I told him about my ongoing respiratory issues. How the more I leaned into my chair, the more my ribs dug into my lungs. And it wasn't like I could do anything about it. Then there was the emotional stress. Jarring movements, people rushing close. Since I couldn't get out of the way, people's quick movements often triggered my adrenaline and affected my breathing.

I told him about my regular visits to the ER. Also about people's comments. "They feel sorry for me and I don't like it. I see it on their faces. Here comes the crooked lady ... One lady in the hallway turned to her husband and said, 'Poor, poor lady.'"

"What did you do?" asked Dr. Dave.

"Well, I know what I wanted to do. I wanted to holler, 'No, I'm not. I'm the most blessed lady around.'"

"Why didn't you?"

I thought for a second. "Because they moved too fast. Okay, you got me there. Maybe I'll say that next time."

He changed the subject. "What's Dr. Clause doing about your breathing?"

"He's given me drugs, nebulizers, and inhalers to open my passageways, and he always tries to stay positive."

Dr. Dave nodded, seemingly satisfied. "Just remember, if you ever need me to talk to the doctors on your behalf, I'm here for you. I can always step in if there's a problem."

Four-Pound Miracle

September 2, 1999

Connor arrived by C-section six weeks ahead of schedule. As I peered into his bassinet, I looked past his tubes and wires. Past the oxygen tube in his nose, the IV in his wrist, and all the chest patches. He might have looked red and blotchy beside the snow-white sheets, but to me, he looked more breathtaking than a double rainbow.

"What a sweetie," I said. "And so tiny. He's practically swimming in that diaper."

The nurse adjusted one of his tubes. "Three pounds, fifteen ounces."

"How long will he have to stay here?"

"Five weeks, maybe six."

I puffed my inhaler, refusing to take my eyes off him. "I brought him a gift." I grabbed the little stuffed lamb from my wheelchair. My hand was still black and blue from my latest IV. How crazy that I had just been home from the ER two days when Connor was born.

The nurse set the lamb beside him. "The perfect touch," she said.

I chuckled. "It's as big as he is." The toy reminded me of my childhood pet lamb, Tiny. We used to always chase each other around the farm.

As I looked at Connor's missing fingers, I remembered what I told Jason and Tara: Get ready. God's giving you a very special baby to take care of.

Seeing the lamb nestled beside him reminded me of Jesus, the Good Shepherd who would always take care of him.

*

"Ema, you look like someone handed you a million bucks," Sandy said. She was Dr. Dave's receptionist.

"Yes, you do," Dr. Dave agreed as he walked out to the waiting area.

"It's better than that," I said. "Someone handed me a four-pound miracle. Connor is home three weeks early from the hospital, and I got to hold him. He's so tiny that he fits perfectly across my arm."

"Well, that explains why you're beaming," Dr. Dave said, rolling my wheelchair the rest of the way into his office. "You know, you're a miracle too, Ema. Just think. You go through crisis after crisis, and you still manage to encourage the rest of us."

"I learn from the best," I said, pulling out a card. "Here ... this is for you."

"What, is it my birthday? Gosh, how did I forget?" He gave me a wink and pulled the card out of the envelope. The picture on the front made him smile: a cat looking into a mirror and seeing the reflection of a lion.

"It reminds me of you," I said. "You help people see better and you give them perspective. We may feel weak, but if we look at ourselves through God's eyes, we see so much more."

"Wise words from a wise lady. So have you thought about getting one?"

"What?"

"A cat."

I laughed. "No ..."

"Well, maybe you should. They're low maintenance and they make great company. Just something you might want to pray about."

"Interesting possibility," I said, smiling.

"So, Ema, tell me … what's going on these days?"

I sighed. "Insurance is forcing me to go to the Cities for a second opinion about my heart. Charlie tried to warn Claire about the drive. He told her how the bumps traumatize my neck and spine and make it hard to breathe. So she knows."

Dr. Dave crossed his arms. "What did she say?"

"She said I had to go anyway."

He shook his head. "I'm sorry."

My throat felt dry as I tried to swallow. "These drives make me nervous because the bumps cause a serious chain reaction in my body. Anything could happen. Which reminds me … I've been meaning to talk to you about something."

"Oh, yeah. About what?"

"If something ever happens to me, would you be able to speak at my funeral?"

He drew back, surprised. "Wow. Ah, I hope it isn't for a long time yet, but sure. Of course I'd be willing. Not only that, but I already know what I'd say."

It was my turn to be surprised. "You do?"

"Why sure … I'll tell them all you're nuts."

I gave him a look and we both cracked up.

Two weeks later, Ellie showed up with a big brown box. "You have some visitors." She set the box on the floor and I heard a little meow.

No way … I hadn't told anybody about my conversation with Dr. Dave.

She lifted the lid and I melted. "Tabbies. Oh, I love them already. Look at their sleepy eyes." I reached in and stroked the smallest one. "Ellie, you're not taking these two little yellow ones. I want these cuties."

She stepped back. "I was kind of hoping you'd say that. We're getting a little overloaded on the farm. Well, it looks like you've got yourself a boy and a girl. Now all you need to do is name them."

I looked at them closely. "This one here looks like a Max, and the little girl looks like a Savannah."

She nodded. "Max and Savannah. I like that."

I stroked their fur. "You kitties make me smile. You're just what the doctor ordered."

Wow. If God cared enough to surprise me with these two little blessings, he'd surely be able to get me to the Cities and back in one piece.

Heart Attack

Sure enough, as we drove north on US Route 52, the bumps waged war on my neck and spine. From her seat behind me, Cathy undid her seat belt and handed me the barf bucket. I emptied out as I often did en route these days, but I still needed to rest my throbbing body.

Bill knew the routine. He'd pull over at the nearest available stop, pull down the ramp, and wheel me out. An hour and a half trip to the Cities easily ended up taking closer to three. While Bill pulled up beside a parked semi, Cathy grabbed my survival pack. That thing came with us everywhere. It included a second barf bucket, disposable washcloths, two water bottles, and a can of 7UP.

Cathy wheeled me over to a grassy area and stuck a straw in the can, while Bill angled himself so we could talk. "How are you doing?"

"Oh, I've been worse," I told him. I'd known Bill for so long that he practically felt like a son. Sometimes, I even joked about adopting him. We made an effort to keep up with each other's kids. He and his wife had even joined us at a couple family reunions. "We R&S drivers fight over you," he told me once. Somehow, I couldn't imagine them fighting over me today.

Cathy tucked my hair behind my ear as cars sped by.

"Shall we pray?" Bill asked. Another oasis in my desert: having a believer for a driver. Bill prayed for me regularly, especially on these longer trips.

"Father, we give you the rest of this ride. Please get us safely to our destination, and please give Ema a strong sense of your love and presence. Amen."

I held my breath as he pushed me back up the ramp. If he didn't position my chair just right, I could hit my head going in. It had happened before, but since then, he'd discovered a special maneuver that kept me safe.

After Bill got me in okay, he needed to park me in the exact spot in the middle. If he parked me too far over, my head could bang into the glass whenever we hit a bump.

But God always took care of me. The last time insurance made me go to the Cities for a second opinion, I managed to get by until our trip back home. We didn't get very far before I had breathing problems. Cathy announced to Brenda, our R&S driver, "Ema needs to go to the ER." We exited as soon as we could and ended up getting lost on a back road somewhere.

"God help us," I prayed. Seconds later, we saw a police car in the rearview mirror. Brenda managed to get the officer's attention, and he led us straight to the ER. I'd lost count on how many times God rescued us like that. Since you can't be rescued unless you're in trouble, I figure we gave God a lot of opportunities to shine hope in our darkness.

Bill centered me behind his seat in the middle and strapped me in. "Thanks," I said. I wondered how long I'd be there before he'd have to pull over and unstrap me again.

Back on the highway, I tried to relax through each blast of pain, but the bumps kept getting worse. Snow and ice wreaked havoc on our Minnesota roads, and we RSD people felt it most.

Cathy repositioned my side pillow. "How's the pain?"

"Sky-high."

She got down on her knees behind me and cupped my head in her hands. It made me think of Psalm 3:3: "But you, LORD, are a shield around me, my glory, the One who lifts my head high."

Keep lifting me, Lord. I need you to lift me ...

The more I struggled to breathe, the more I retreated into my secret prayer place. Cathy knew where I went, just like she knew when I needed to feel Jesus extra close.

Somehow we got there. But as I sat in the doctor's office, Cathy stepped back. "Your face!" She pulled out a mirror, and sure enough, my face and neck were bright red and covered with white hives. My hands and ankles had them too, and I struggled to breathe. Forget all my scheduled tests. I had to go right to the ER.

As Bill pushed the wheelchair down the hall, I wondered what Claire would think if she saw me now. Would she regret sending me here?

"I'll take you in," a short blonde nurse said.

Cathy spoke up. "We need to make sure the door's wide enough."

"No problem." And she led us straight to a room where a tall nurse waited with a needle. "We need to give her this shot of epinephrine."

As the needle went in, the tall nurse signaled to the blonde, "Let's get her in bed."

Cathy stepped between them. "No, don't. Ema stays in her wheelchair. We can't compromise her spine." She was right. The last time nurses tried to put me in a bed, I felt like a human wishbone. Hands pressed into my rib cage, stealing my breath. I literally felt ripped apart, like my upper torso had been detached from my lower torso. It's a wonder they didn't crack my spine.

The blonde nurse looked at Cathy like she'd lost her mind. "What? We can't put her in bed?"

Cathy shook her head. "It would traumatize her spine. Oh, and it says so right here." She pulled out the doctor's form, and the tall nurse squinted to look. The form informed doctors that I had advanced reflex sympathetic dystrophy. The words in bold letters couldn't be missed: "DO NOT remove Ema McKinley from her wheelchair which would be harmful to her general health because of this pain syndrome."

"Okay," the nurse said. "I guess we'll just move the bed against the wall and keep her wheelchair in the middle of the room."

As they shuffled around, I felt like a misfit, because that's what I was. They busied themselves taking my vitals—my blood pressure, pulse, and temperature. Suddenly their faces got serious and the blonde nurse quickly and quietly pointed something out to the doctor.

"Hook her up to a heart monitor." He ordered an ECG, and the next thing I knew, they had electrodes on me. "Looks like a mild heart attack," the doctor said. "We'll do some blood tests."

Heart attack? What next, I wondered? While everybody talked about my heart, blood pressure, and blood cell count, I closed my thoughts in around Jesus. Their tests ran late into the night. Then I sat in the dark like a broken mannequin in the middle of the room. I prayed for Brady, Connor, Ellie, and even Eddie. I couldn't forget to thank God for church friends who could peek in on Max and Savannah. I even prayed for the folks at the insurance company, who, by now, could see for themselves that I truly had heart problems.

I meditated on the words from Deuteronomy 8:2–3. "Remember how the LORD your God led you all the way in the wilderness these forty years, to humble and test you in order to know what was in your heart, whether or not you would keep his commands. He humbled you, causing you to hunger and then feeding you with manna, which neither you nor your ancestors had known, to teach you that man does not live on bread alone but on every word that comes from the mouth of the LORD."

Lord, I want to pass each test. I want to be humble and keep all your commands. I want to love your words more and more, just like I love you. Thank you for being the light when I don't see where I'm going. Thank you for teaching me that I can always trust you, no matter what.

＊

After four days in the hospital, they told me I was stable enough to go home.

"Good to know I'm stable," I said.

The doctor stayed serious. "Because of what happened on your ride up here, we'd like to give you a shot of Ativan to relax you on the way home. It should also help you fall asleep."

Naturally, the sleep part didn't happen, but the shot sure made me super groggy. I'd never felt like such a zombie. Strange. My mind felt a thousand miles away. Almost like I was somebody else.

Oddly, the drive home felt easy as pie. Even the bumps didn't bother me. Why hadn't they given me this stuff before? In the whole hour and a half, I didn't even need the barf bucket. I stayed half comatose all the way home. And then, shortly afterward, the sobs ripped out of me.

Dark Cloud

October 6, 1999

The ring of the phone vibrated in my ears. What was wrong with people these days?

"Hello!"

"Ema, it's your dad. I need to come over."

"I want to be alone," I mumbled.

"Ema, please ... Cathy and Ellie told me you haven't been the same since you got home from the Cities. We're worried, and I'd like to talk to you for a bit."

My heart ripped. "I can't. I need to go."

Half an hour later, I heard a knock on the door, followed by Cathy's muffled voice. "Open up."

"What do you want?"

"Ellie and I need to talk with you. We want to help you."

"No, thanks. You can't do anything anyway. I just want to be alone."

I knew I was rude, but I didn't care. I couldn't. Confusion sprayed graffiti all over my brain. My whole life felt like an old, wrung-out, twisted, good-for-nothing cloth.

I flicked on the stereo, but it sounded like a bunch of noise, pulsing, grating, digging into my ears like fingernails on a chalkboard.

Savannah and Max pawed at my foot and tried rubbing on my leg for attention. "Go away!" I couldn't even stand the sight of them.

Their meows got under my skin. Who gave them the right to be so demanding?

My face felt flat. Sagged under a weight I couldn't lift no matter how hard I tried. My frown pressed deep, falling, falling. And my mind right along with it ... into a lifetime of sad, grievous memories.

I thought about when we moved to the house on the hill. We had Douse, our big, beautiful black-and-white sheepdog. Douse loved people so much that whenever anybody visited the farm, he followed their car up the lane. He had so much energy. When we went to a family reunion at Grandma and Grandpa Reeves' house, my dad decided to tie his chain to the doghouse so he wouldn't jump on anybody while we were gone.

We had a great time, but I looked forward to coming home to Douse. As we drove up the lane, we saw something that made our hearts stop. Douse. He was hanging upside down over his doghouse. The image of his dangling dead body stamped deep in my brain.

Bad dog for trying to jump over your doghouse when your chain got caught.

I thought about how Grandma Reeves died a couple months later. I'd never been to a funeral so I didn't know what to expect. Boy, did I miss Grandma Reeves something fierce. And what I wouldn't do to hear her play the piano, sing a hymn, and laugh one last time.

The church had been full. So with eight people in our family, I got separated from my parents and ended up sitting by myself—just two thin rows away from Grandma's open casket. I couldn't tear my wide eyes from her motionless body, her chalky face, and slicked-back hair.

Afterward, when we went to Grandma's farm for the reception, I dashed off and hid in her closet with her skirts, sweaters, and shoes. Sobbing, I breathed in and out, trying to savor her smells.

"Ema. Where are you?" my mother and aunt called.

I didn't say anything. I didn't want to come out. I just wanted to keep breathing.

When they found me, their faces looked flushed, not like Grandma's. They crouched down beside me. They looked serious.

"Don't cry," my aunt said. "It's okay. Grandma's in heaven now. She's all better. Please come out so we can talk."

I shook my head adamantly. "No. I want to be alone."

Just like I now told everybody who came to my townhome. Go away. Leave me alone. Except this new sudden blackness loomed a thousand shades darker.

After three days of the darkness, I decided to venture to my deck, but my wheelchair kept catching on the threshold.

"Stupid chair!" I yelled. I didn't care if the neighbors heard me. I just wanted to get out. But the more I tried, the more I got stuck. I banged angry fists on the wall and couldn't stop sobbing. Why did everything have to fall apart? It was wrong. All wrong. *I* was wrong.

Darkness kept closing in. I hated it, this thick, ugly shade being pulled over my world.

Wouldn't it be easier not to feel? Everyone's lives would be better without me.

I gave my chair another yank and that did it. I finally made it outside into the sunshine. So much for improving my mood. It did absolutely nothing. I stared at my big pot of flowers, at the two butterfly decorations on the side of the house, at the noisy children in the field. And a slow coldness crept over me like I'd never known. It bit into me, this lonely desperation ... and it terrified me.

A loud cry escaped my throat. What was happening? Something wasn't right, and I couldn't figure it out. But I couldn't stay in this dungeon.

I'm better than this, I told myself. I'm stronger than this. Where was that strength I'd always known? Oh, I hated this feeling. Hated this evil eating me alive, taking me lower and lower.

Finally, the faintest flicker of light broke through my thoughts—and I knew what I had to do. I had to reach for it with praise and thanksgiving. I had to stir it up and spill it out.

Thank you, God, that you're in this coldness, this darkness, this hell on earth.

In that sliver of a moment, I felt the tiniest edge of my shade start to lift.

Thank you, God, for family, for friends, for my wheelchair, for this body, for this trial. Even thank you for bringing at least a smidgen of good out of every single horrible thing that has ever happened to me.

Just then I felt something. Jesus. His presence. I felt the weight of his hand on my shoulder . . .

Jesus . . . you're here.

The most beautiful peace fell on me as he spoke into my spirit:

"Ema, I've always been here. I've never left you."

His words of truth brought warmth, melting the wax of my heaviness.

A song crept into my thinking: "Put on the garment of praise for the spirit of heaviness."

Yes, Lord, I do praise you. You are mighty. You are my everything. All I ever need.

I wanted to keep praising him. In my deepest darkness, he'd reached down to me and shown me how much stronger he is. He helped me find him again—even though he'd never really left me in the first place.

When I told Dr. Dave what happened, his eyes widened.

"Did you know that one of the rare side effects of that medicine is severe depression?"

I shook my head. "Nobody mentioned it."

"Ema, it normally takes people several months to come out of that same level of depression. You got over it in three days. That's unheard of."

I didn't know what to say. Even with all my RSD battles, I'd never been depressed. Sure, I'd had my down days, but nothing like this. It seemed strange that a drug could take me down so far, so fast. And it felt equally strange that I could get over it so fast. From what Dr. Dave said, that in itself was a miracle.

He threw up his hands. "See, I told you you're a tough old bird."

It felt so good to smile I didn't ever want to stop. Even when other thoughts nagged beneath the surface. What if God hadn't intervened? And what about my cats? I'd sunk so deep in my pit that I hadn't bothered to give them any fresh food for three whole days. Just thinking about it made me feel sick and ashamed.

Don't go there, I told myself. God didn't want me to camp on the negative side. Only Satan did.

I remembered how Jesus spoke to the Pharisees in John 10:10: "The thief comes only to steal and kill and destroy; I have come that they may have life, and have it to the full."

Okay, Lord ... am I living life to the full yet?

Child Ambassador

December 2000

When Connor was fifteen months old, the March of Dimes chose him to be their child ambassador for the year, which meant I'd have the privilege of being the spokesperson for the family. My heart danced.

You've done it again, Lord. You've given me another fun purpose. And how perfect that it should happen at the end of the year 2000. A special event for a special year. What an honor. And it will stretch through the next year as well. Thanks for the blessing!

Shortly after I heard the news, I asked Tara if she wanted to brainstorm. "If we put our heads together," I said, "I'm sure we could come up with some fabulous fund-raiser ideas. And if you're okay with it, I'd like to include Brady, now that he's five."

"He'd love it. Hey, Brady. Come here for a minute." Brady skipped into the kitchen with a toy car in his hand. "Brady, would you like to help Grandma raise money to help handicapped kids?"

He bobbed his head up and down.

"Oh, good," I said. "You'll be a fabulous help."

As we gathered around the table, we tossed ideas back and forth. It didn't take long before God gave me a good one. A gem. "We could buy piggy banks and set them up at local gas stations. People always have change. I bet they'd donate to the March of Dimes in a heartbeat. What do you think, Brady? Is that a good idea?"

His eyes lit up. "Yup. That's what I want to do. I want to get piggy

146

banks. And we could buy boy ones for the boys and girl ones for the girls."

"Absolutely," I said.

So we drove to Michaels, the arts and crafts store, and filled our cart with dozens of piggy banks and spools of colored ribbon. At home, Brady helped tie pink bows around the heads of the girl piggy banks and the blue bows around the ones for boys. I loved doing things together.

When the time came to stop at gas stations, I couldn't have been more animated. We gave each of them two pigs and a poster that featured our very own Connor as the child ambassador. I admit, the mission nearly drained me dry, but it helped to focus on the good we were doing.

Because of Connor's new role, we had a smorgasbord of events to attend. Good thing Connor didn't mind. He ate up the attention as if he was born for it. People beamed and fussed all over him. They held him on their laps and played with him. It made me thankful all over again that they chose him.

One of the events we participated in was the fund-raiser car wash. While cars got sudsy and clowns got goofy, I talked to everyone willing to listen about the organization and what we stood for.

As we got closer to our big annual walkathon, the coordinator asked me to help with something I'd never done before. Radio interviews. Of course, I readily agreed. How hard could it be? All I'd have to do was speak from the heart.

"We need more money for research," I told the radio audience. "We're blessed to have an opportunity to help these babies before they're born. My grandson was born with deformities. It might be too late for him, but it's certainly not too late for others. And that's why we're having this big walkathon in the first place. If we raise more money, we can conduct more research. So we definitely welcome your involvement. You can either walk or just make pledges. But you need to know that every bit helps. We can all make a difference for those unborn babies and their mothers."

April 28, 2001

When the big day finally arrived, my heart leaped as much as the excited kids. I loved this walkathon event, especially because of all the good memories I'd collected over the years.

Back in my day care days, I went the whole distance on Rollerblades. I'd stick a toddler in my backpack carrier and away I'd go. I'd even rotate children along the way. I'd skate the whole seven miles with energy to spare.

Today, however, I could barely hold little Connor for a thirty-second newspaper photo. Goodness, I wished I could do more, but such was life. And I wouldn't let it get me down. The Lord had always been faithful to me. The least I could do was focus on my blessings and keep moving forward.

When the guy blew the whistle, Tara and Jason kicked off with Connor in the stroller.

"See you at the finish line!" I hollered. "Have fun!"

I didn't care who pushed my wheelchair. I started with George, the manager from Kmart. But somewhere along the route, he handed me off to somebody else — kind of like what I used to do when I switched toddlers.

On the final stretch, Bruce took over. I didn't know him quite as well as some of the others, but boy, did he ever put a lot of thunder into it. I guess I got so caught up in the sights and sounds with everybody racing around me that I never for a second imagined something bad might happen.

Until we hit a bump.

My upper torso flew off the steel platform attachment. And it came down again with such a crash that I felt it in my bones. Cracked ribs.

If Bruce had seen the look on my face, he would have stopped blabbering. "We're really flying, Ema. This is great."

Searing pain ripped into me. This wasn't the first time I'd cracked my ribs. It happened another time when one of the R&S drivers hit a big bump in the Kmart parking lot. Back then, everybody knew about it right away. This time, poor Bruce didn't have a clue—and I didn't want to tell him. What would it accomplish besides make him feel like a heel? We were almost at the end.

Hang in there, I told myself.

Climbing the next hill, I could see it. The finish line. It looked more glorious than a sunset.

Just then we hit another bump. Breathe, I told myself. You'll soon be home.

But I'd forgotten about the press. A middle-aged man ran over like he'd been waiting for me all day. While my cracked ribs stabbed and throbbed, he stuck a television camera in my face.

"Congratulations, Ema. You did it." He turned to the camera. "We're talking with this year's spokesperson for the child ambassador. Ema McKinley. Ema, can you tell us what a great time you had on the walk this year?"

I didn't usually paste on smiles—except in emergencies.

Okay, here we go, Lord . . .

I sucked in a breath. "The annual March of Dimes walk has always been one of my very favorite events. Volunteers look forward to it all year long. Personally, all I can really say about it right now is . . . Wow. Every year is unique and oh so full of surprises."

A week and a half later, Ellie wheeled me to the pharmacy to pick up more pain medication. As she pushed me by the shelves along the far wall, one of the clerks stopped us. "Mind if I talk to you for a second?"

"Sure. That's fine," I said.

She moved closer. "I've seen you come in here quite a bit. I know what kind of medications you're on, so I imagine you're going through something really horrible. But every time I see you, you're smiling. You look so happy to be alive. Well, a couple weeks ago, I went through something really horrible myself." She got quiet. "I actually swallowed some pills and tried to end my life."

I grabbed her hand. "You didn't!"

She nodded regretfully. "There's more. After I took the pills, I saw the newspaper with that picture of you and your grandson for the March of Dimes walkathon. It really opened my eyes. The first thing I thought was: I know her. I know what she goes through. Then all of a sudden I realized ... what am I doing? I don't have it so bad. If this dear woman can go through this kind of incredible suffering and still find a purpose, well, maybe I can too. So you know what I did next? I grabbed the phone and called 911. And that's why I'm still here today. I just had to tell you ... Thanks. You saved my life."

Tears rolled down my face as I squeezed her hand. "Thank you for sharing that. I'll remember to pray for you."

The whole drive home I couldn't stop praising the Lord. Even through the bumps on the road, fresh waves of thankfulness washed over me.

Jesus, thank you for stepping in and sparing this beautiful young lady. You want to use my pain for good, don't you? I can see it, and this is just another proof. Well, you know what, God? If my pain helps others, I think I'd even say it's worth it.

On my deck back at home, I pondered 1 Peter 4:1–2: "Therefore, since Christ suffered in his body, arm yourselves also with the same attitude, because whoever suffers in the body is done with sin. As a result, they do not live the rest of their earthly lives for evil human desires, but rather for the will of God."

I knew Jesus had taken care of my sins on the cross and that I didn't need to do anything to earn it. So what did this verse mean then? I didn't exactly know. All I knew was I wanted to be like Jesus more than ever. Full surrender—right down to every last breath.

Here I am again, Lord, offering myself to you. Take this deformed and bent body. Take my whole life. My everything. Mold me exactly as you want me—into your perfect image.

Cancer

February 2003

Dr. Bengston, my wise upper-extremity doctor, looked at me sympathetically. "So the pain's gotten worse again?"

I'd been through so much with this doctor over the years. How many times had he heard me try to gauge the pain? I'd lost count, but I'm sure it had to be a bit depressing.

"Have you ever heard of thalidomide?" he asked.

I stiffened. "Isn't that the drug they used to give to pregnant mothers? The one they made illegal because it caused birth defects?"

He nodded. "They took thalidomide off the market for a while, but a few years ago they made it legal for people suffering with RSD. It helps with the pain, so it could be a good complement with your morphine."

I hated to ask the next question, but it came with the territory. "What are the side effects?"

His eyebrows arched up. "Weight gain's a common one. A lot of people can't handle the fatigue either. That's often why people go off it, because it makes them want to sleep all the time."

"Boy, I wish it would have that effect on me."

Naturally, I didn't like the idea of gaining weight any more than the next person. But I'd sure been down that road before. With so many prescriptions firing at me, I'd experienced it all. Some of them had shrunk me right back down again. But overall, the more my RSD advanced and the more I took drugs, the more my weight shot up. Who knows ... maybe I'd end up looking like one big curve rolling into another. Still, I'd do just about anything to ease the pain.

As Ellie wheeled me into Dr. Dave's waiting room, I knew we'd have to talk and pray about my new medicine. Whether I had good news or bad news, Dr. Dave was always the best listener.

Sandy, his sweet receptionist, stood as soon as she saw me.

When I saw her puffy eyes, my stomach went weak. "What's wrong?"

She shook her head. "Ema, I'm sorry. I didn't have time to call you."

A patch of dry skin on the knuckle of my club fist itched something fierce. "Call me about what?"

"Oh ... I've never had to do this before."

"Do what? What's going on?"

"It's Dr. Dave. I need to cancel all his appointments."

My heart pounded. "Why?"

She drew in a breath. "He has cancer, Ema. I'm sorry. He just found out."

The air in the waiting room got sucked out by an invisible vacuum. How could it be? I'd just seen him the previous week and he looked fine. Cancer? Not Dr. Dave. No! Of all my doctors, he'd helped me more than anybody. He was my rock. Surely he'd get better. He had to.

I tried to clear my throat. "What do the doctors say?"

"It's stage four leukemia. They've already started him on chemotherapy. It doesn't look good."

I stared at his office window — into the darkness. He'd taped the card I gave him on the glass, the one with the picture of the cat looking in a mirror and seeing a lion.

I left the building in a daze, praying with everything in me. *Please, oh please, fit healing into your plan for him, Lord.*

✳

Four weeks later, when I was in my office, the phone rang and I grabbed it.

"Ema? It's Sandy."

"How's Dr. Dave?"

Her pause made the phone feel sweaty in my hand. "Hello? Are you still there?"

"I'm ... very sorry," she said slowly. "He's gone."

It didn't hit me until I got to the funeral home a few days later. The place was packed as I inched to the open casket. Voices pressed in as people shared: "Dave was such a pillar at his church. So well loved." "What a wonderful man." "He was always so real."

I sucked in a shallow breath as I glanced at his vacant body. The leukemia had literally shrunk him. And because the chemo had taken his hair, he now wore a toupee.

When I saw others grieving, tears streamed down my face. I thought of Dr. Dave's listening heart. His kind, loving words. I was his TOB, his tough old bird. My chest soon heaved into sobs. When I wasn't expecting it, a hand came down on my shoulder. I jumped.

"It's okay," Dr. Dave's wife said. "He isn't hurting anymore." We hugged and I ignored the lump in my throat. "He thought the world of you, Ema. Your strength in the Lord taught him so much."

"Thanks." I managed to smile. She stood beside me as I glanced at the empty shell of his body.

He'd agreed to speak at my funeral. So much for that idea. Why did he have to be the first to go? It didn't make sense. Here I was, all bent in my wheelchair, and now he was probably dancing his heart out—free from disease and hardship. Gazing into the eyes of our Savior.

The last thing I wanted was to see another psychologist—someone who'd make me revisit the accident and reopen my heart. No, thank you. Because nobody could replace Dr. Dave. It wouldn't be possible.

A few months after the funeral, however, Sandy called. "I think we found you a new psychologist."

"Oh, I don't know ..."

"I realize it's a bit soon, but I think Dr. Cindy Smith would be a great match for you. I know it's scary, but think about it. It wouldn't hurt to visit at least once. I'll even go with you."

The more she talked, the more my resistance broke down. "Okay," I said finally. "I suppose one little visit wouldn't hurt."

Later that same day, I sat across from a young, attractive gray-haired woman with bright, compassionate eyes and a smooth voice.

"Great to meet you," she said. "I'm so sorry to hear about Dr. Dave. He was such a great guy."

"You knew him?"

She nodded.

Okay, I thought to myself. At least we have a great place to start.

Dr. Cindy and I spent the next forty-five minutes talking about our mutual appreciation for Dr. Dave as well as our love for the Lord. I found it quite healing. And the more we talked, the more I felt my first little flickers of trust. Clearly, Dr. Cindy was someone I could see myself turning to in the difficult days ahead.

Out of Oxygen

Fall 2003

One busy day, after returning home from a long string of doctor appointments, my breathing became so tight that I had to use my nebulizer and inhalers.

"They aren't working," Ellie said. "She's going down fast."

Cathy went into autopilot. "I'll make the phone calls."

Of course, she couldn't just call 911. Minnesota state law required that all ambulance patients be transported on a gurney. And since strapping me down would never work with my crooked spine, she had to also call R&S.

Within minutes, I heard the sirens. A police car, fire truck, and ambulance were somewhere in front of my little townhome, with the R&S van right behind them.

The men came in and tried to unpry me from the table. Fighting for air, I'd curled my fingers around the wood in gripping panic. The kind of panic that soaks your clothes clear through.

After they unstuck me, they started an IV. "Let's go," one of them said. The kitchen door swung open and they hurried me down the ramp. A few neighbors formed a little cluster near the road.

Two paramedics, one from the fire truck and one from the ambulance, left their vehicles and partners and hopped inside the R&S van beside me. Several paramedics were used to this. They knew the routine. Marnie, one of my newer R&S drivers, did not.

"Follow the ambulance," ordered a paramedic. "They'll clear the way. And ignore the red traffic lights."

"I don't know about this," she said nervously. "I don't want anyone dying on my shift."

Lights flashed and sirens blared as they rushed me to the hospital. Somewhere along the ride, I must have thrashed my arm because something happened to my IV. Blood squirted out all over the place.

After they cleaned me up, one of the guys repositioned my mask. Normally, I would think of the burn marks it would leave, but not today. My airways constricted tighter and tighter. I could tell this was more serious than other times. As my fingers went numb and the clouds and treetops began to blur, I wondered if I'd even make it to the hospital.

"Hang in there," a paramedic said. "We're pulling in now."

I gasped for air—hungry for every last trace of it. Heaven must be close. I could feel it. Heaven, Jesus, angels ...

"The LORD is my shepherd, I lack nothing. He makes me lie down in green pastures ..."

Somewhere behind all my pain and breathlessness, I felt peace. I knew where I was going. It was only a matter of time.

A doctor grabbed my wheelchair and rushed me inside. "Quick. We need a room where she'll fit."

"Neurology!" someone yelled.

As soon as they got me in, they connected me to a machine. Daddy, Ellie, and Cathy gathered around. My breath came out in short, shallow gusts.

"We need to get her down," said the doctor.

Cathy stepped in front of him and stretched out her arms. "Ema stays in her wheelchair. She doesn't come out."

He jolted his head in frustration. "We need to get her down so we can help her."

"No," Cathy insisted. "We have paperwork."

A nurse spoke up. "Oxygen's in the low forties and going down fast."

"Call a code," snapped the doctor.

While everyone spun into high gear, I began to shut down. With everything in me, I pulled for air. I didn't flail or convulse. I did the only thing I could do: I sat there. I asked the Lord, *How much longer?*

" . . . He leads me beside quiet waters, he refreshes my soul. He guides me along the right paths for his name's sake."

Voices competed in the hallway. Sounds blurred, instruments clanged, feet stirred.

"I love you," Daddy said in my ear.

I wanted to say the same thing back: *I love you, Daddy.* But air restricted me — suffocating, tightening, pulling me away . . .

Daddy lightly touched my hand. *"Lord Jesus, may Ema feel your arms around her."*

"Hurry," the doctor said. "We need to intubate. Move! If we don't get this tube down her throat, we're gonna lose her."

"No!" Cathy said. "No tube."

"What do you mean no tube?" the doctor yelled.

"Ema's wishes," Cathy said. "Look, I have them right here on this form. Do not resuscitate."

"Listen, if we don't open up her passageway, she won't make it. As it is, she only has four or five minutes — at most."

Four or five minutes? The words echoed in my throat, rang in my brain, a beacon of light. Soon, so very soon I'd be dancing with Jesus . . .

"Even though I walk through the darkest valley, I will fear no evil, for you are with me . . ."

Ellie got down on her knees. She got so close I felt her breath in my ear. "Ema, are you sure you want a DNR? Are you sure you want to keep your wishes?"

"Yes." I mouthed the word.

"Okay, then," Ellie said, stepping back, satisfied.

Doctors and nurses grumbled in frustration and slowly started backing away. They weren't in my shoes. They didn't know the constant pain I was in. If they had, they would have been happy for me.

Daddy and Cathy and Ellie stepped closer, treasuring each second of our last moments together. I closed my eyes.

Soon, Jesus . . . I'm coming home soon . . .

Suddenly, a loud commanding voice broke into my thoughts.

Ema, breathe!

I knew that voice. It was the same voice I'd heard through all those years.

Jesus!

In a sliver of a moment, I let out one of the loudest, biggest gasps I'd ever breathed in my entire life. And I went from drowning to floating.

Doctors and nurses rushed back over with shock on their faces. One squinted at the monitor. Another one rushed to the door to call the others. That's when I learned that they had a whole team waiting in the hallway.

"Quick, get in here," the doctor shouted. "You've got to see this!"

I heard a rumble of questions about what happened and saw the doctor try to explain. "I don't know. Her passageway just opened up on its own."

I smiled up at them. "I guess it wasn't my time."

Confusion and relief traded places with fear and panic. Eyes clouded and doctors looked at each other as if to say, *What next?*

"Well, I guess I can go home now," I said.

One of the doctors stifled a laugh. "Ah . . . I don't think that would be a good idea. You just about died a few minutes ago. You should at least stay overnight so we can monitor you."

"But why? I'm alive and breathing now, aren't I? I'm fine."

A nurse rested her hand on my shoulder. "Yes, that's wonderful and amazing, but we think it's wise to monitor you and make sure everything's okay. Would that work?"

I hesitated. "Ah, I suppose," I said. "Go ahead and do your tests."

Of course, everything looked great. At least as great as could be expected. I was back to my normal abnormal self.

I had a follow-up visit the next day with Dr. Clause. Before I was wheeled out of the hall and into his office, a voice called out from behind me. "Hey! If it isn't Lazarus back from the dead."

"Dr. Clause!" I exclaimed. "You heard!"

He caught up with us. "Big news travels fast."

Man, I loved the joy on his face. But even more, I loved being called Lazarus. What a hoot. I'd been called a slew of things in my life, but that was a first. Lazarus. I almost giggled when I pictured him all wrapped up tight in one of those long, thick strands of cloth, all mummy-like.

It was quite flattering actually. Jesus loved Lazarus so much that he wept over him. Goodness, the man played a key role in Scripture. Jesus used his broken life to show us what would one day happen to each one of us.

Sores

Spring 2004

Dr. David Bell, my new primary-care doctor, walked in, his eyes sparkling beneath his thick head of brown hair. "How's it going?"

I gave him a stiff laugh, partly because I didn't want to tell him I had another crisis. "You know those awful sores I've had in different places? Well, they've gotten much worse. Now they're all over my legs. A real mess."

He pursed his lips. "Let's take a look."

He couldn't have been prepared for the sight. What had started off months ago as a few simple red splotches had now morphed into a raging sea of gruesomeness. I couldn't stand it. The sores were as painful as they were weepy.

Dr. Bell didn't hide his concern. And he sent me right to Dr. Clark Otley, a dermatologist.

Dr. Otley was a soft-spoken, gentle man, especially when it came to my sores. He showed genuine empathy. "Your right leg is infected, Ema. We need to start wrapping it regularly and teaching your caregivers how to do it as well."

"Okay," I said absently. As to what would become of this, only the Lord knew.

Cathy and Ellie watched closely as Dr. Otley smothered my leg in thick Vaseline before wrapping it in several thick layers of gauze. "You'll have to do this every couple hours," he instructed.

I couldn't think of anything more disgusting to ask somebody to do for me. But, bless their hearts, the two rolled up their sleeves and did it without complaining. But how sad that after just a couple hours of slathering and wrapping, the wetness seeped clear through! It almost seemed like my leg wouldn't stop crying, and it was trying to pull me right along with it!

Because this was so time consuming, Cathy and Ellie trained some of my other friends how to dress the sores too. Out of the kindness of their hearts, Cathy, Mariah, and Janet all took turns coming over to help.

"Don't scratch it," they reminded me. The sores itched like crazy, but I mostly learned the hard way not to mess with them. Of course, seeing my skin slough off in big, thick scales when I scratched was a good reminder not to.

My caregivers and friends made a full day of it, but I couldn't see asking them to do it all through the night. That would be too much. So after the last person wrapped me around midnight, I had her place a tall stack of towels on the second desk in my office. That desk was at the perfect level to rest my head between leg treatments. All night long, I used towel after towel, blotting and soaking until I was surrounded. Invaded by a big heap of dirty laundry that did nothing more than eat up my endless rain of fluids.

In addition to this time-consuming, gross-beyond-words leg problem, I still had to deal with all the pain. Weeks of these itchy, weepy sores turned into months. And just to make life more interesting, I still had respiratory issues. It wasn't easy to stay positive because I knew the truth: if something didn't change, I'd be in trouble.

September 2004

When Dr. Otley got down at my level, I could tell from his serious expression that he had something important to say.

"The Minnesota Dermatological Society would like you to attend one of their key seminars. A wide variety of doctors gather together to exchange information about highly unusual skin disorders. And your sores qualify."

"Just curious," I said, "but what good would it do?"

"Well, for one thing the research could help us find more information about your condition. On top of that, it could help others."

"Count me in then," I told him.

So that's how I ended up in a tiny room surrounded by five eager doctors clutching notebooks with gloved hands.

"We've done all our preliminary research," an older one said. His white hair matched his beard. "Thanks again for being available for our study."

"You're welcome, I think."

"Let's take a look," a doctor said in an Australian accent.

A hush fell over the room as, layer by layer, he pulled back the gauze from my mummy-like leg. I thought back to how I appreciated being associated with Lazarus. It seemed like a lifetime ago. As soon as the doctor peeled off the last layer of gauze and dropped it in the bin, everyone gasped. I felt the pain in their faces as my raw, weepy flesh stared back at them.

The Australian doctor didn't have to look close to make a simple observation because even my toes looked sick. Every day they'd been growing darker and more discolored.

He jotted something on his clipboard and stepped back. "These sores are worldwide rare," he said. "I've never seen them progress to this level."

"I'm glad to hear they're rare," I said, "because I sure wouldn't wish them on anybody."

A doctor stepped forward with a bucket. "We're going to stick this under your heel to collect your fluids. Then we'll send them to Disease Control and tell you what they find."

"Go ahead," I said. "Collect away."

The doctors exchanged looks as my fluids dripped all the way down my leg and slid off my heel into the bucket.

The two women looked grief-stricken and glazed as they dabbed their eyes, trying to hide their tears. "Poor thing," one of them said. "And she's had this for several months."

The other gal shook her head. "I know. I can't even imagine."

I felt a lot of emotions as I took it all in. Personally, I'd never felt such a strong connection with my old buddy Job—my Bible friend who endured all those painful, itchy sores.

The Australian said, "On a scale of one to ten, how would you rate the itch?"

"It varies somewhere between ten and twenty."

The doctor who had placed the bucket stepped back so we could make eye contact. "Does it help to eat certain foods or vitamins?"

"I can only take protein drinks."

The Australian clasped his gloved hands together. "In other cases of RSD sores, patients find a certain amount of relief by smoking marijuana. Has anyone ever suggested this to you?"

I laughed. "No, and I'm not really interested, thank you."

"What about horse chestnut extract? Ever tried that?"

I scrunched my nose. "Horseradish?"

"No, not horseradish. Horse chestnut extract. It's helped in some cases."

"Hmm," I mused. "I'll be sure to keep that in mind."

The following week when I sat in Dr. Otley's office, my fluids had already been to Disease Control and back.

"Goodness, those things get around faster than I do."

Dr. Otley stayed serious. "Your results are quite puzzling. Nobody has ever seen your types of infections before."

"Wow, I stumped them. So where does this leave us then?"

He crossed his arms. "Well, we've been giving you different types of antibiotics, but since you don't seem to be responding to them yet, I think we're going to have to raise your dose."

That sounded all too familiar. "Um, something else has been bothering me. I've kind of been having sharp pains behind my right knee. You can't quite see anything, but it really hurts. It's probably nothing, but ..."

"Well, let's take a look."

He knelt down and looked at it a little longer than I expected.

"Do you see anything?"

Concern wrinkled his brow as he stood up. "I think we need to order an ultrasound."

At my next Dr. Otley appointment, five doctors walked in. Two doctors wouldn't have surprised me, because I was used to seeing people shadow Dr. Otley. They all wanted to check out the crooked lady with the sores. But four extra doctors? Now that was a red flag.

Dr. Otley adjusted his glasses. "I don't know how to say this."

How many times had I heard that phrase. "Just tell me."

He bit down on his lip. "Your condition has become life-threatening. You've had these sores for several months. You now have three different types of infections. And on top of that, your black toes couldn't look more dead. And to make matters worse, you now have several blood clots in your leg."

I stared at him. "Blood clots?"

"I'm afraid so. And if they travel to your heart, they could be fatal. To be frank, these infections could be fatal too—if we don't get them under control."

"What are you suggesting?"

He ran a hand through his hair. "I think we need to amputate your right leg."

The room got quiet. Nobody moved.

"Amputate my leg?" My voice sounded as wooden as it felt. With my left leg permanently locked under my wheelchair, my right leg was the only one I could depend on. I used it to push myself around at night. I had tried a motorized chair, but the vibration charged up my spine and neck with such a quick buzz of pain that I couldn't stand it. I owed my little bit of mobility to that limited right leg.

I took a deep breath and blew it out slowly. There it was, that same old fear trying to shake the bananas out of my tree. I reached for more faith and found it. It came like a little tossing of leaves.

"I'll pray about it."

"Okay, but you need to tell us as soon as possible. It could be a matter of life and death."

I wanted nothing more than to go home and have a good, long cry. The problem was, I desperately needed more gauze from the pharmacy. Gauze had become a basic staple. Kind of as important as toilet paper.

Ellie moved me slowly toward the counter. She knew how much I dreaded coming here. We both did. Every time we filled a prescription, the clerks had to call insurance for approval. And none of the clerks or pharmacists wanted to talk to Claire Rhodes. Whenever I got to the counter, they shuffled to the other side. They busied themselves with their products and paperwork, hoping somebody else would deal with me instead.

A younger gal stepped up to the counter. "May I help you?"

"Yes, please. I need this prescription filled." As I handed it to her, I almost wanted to apologize. Then, when she picked up the phone, I tensed.

She had time to say only a few words before she covered her hand over the receiver and leaned over, red-faced. "Ema? Claire Rhodes wants to talk to you."

Ellie and I exchanged looks. Through all the times we'd done this, Claire had never asked to talk to me. Why now? Why today?

Ellie took the phone and handed it to me. "Hello?"

"Ema McKinley?"

"Yes."

"I'd like to have a word with you. May I ask what's going on with all these gauze prescriptions? I've never heard of anybody needing such an impossible amount. Don't you think it's a bit excessive? I mean, when's it going to stop?"

I could hardly breathe. "You don't know what you're saying, Claire. Because if you did, you wouldn't say it. For one thing, just today the doctors told me they want to amputate my leg. To cut it off. So if you really want to know what I'm dealing with, that's what."

She sighed loudly. "All I know is you're costing us *way* too much money. It's a crying shame. It's getting ridiculous."

My hand shook as I handed the phone back to Ellie.

When I returned home, Savannah must have sensed my pain because she walked away from her cat food and jumped on my lap. "Thanks, girl," I said, stroking her fur. The house was quiet except for her purrs. I wanted it that way so I could dive into my secret place with Jesus. He and I needed to have a good long talk about my leg and its future.

I closed my eyes and imagined him beside me. He was there, after all.

Breathing deep, I decided to take him up on James 1:5: "If any of you lacks wisdom, you should ask God, who gives generously to all without finding fault, and it will be given to you."

Father, I'm not just asking. I'm begging. Please show me what to do about my leg.

All through the night, using towel after towel on my sores, I poured out my heart to God. As I dabbed and blotted, I thought of the woman washing Jesus' feet. Those Pharisees sure got all uptight with Jesus: "If you knew who she really was, you never would have let her touch your feet!"

167

Jesus knew exactly who she was. A prostitute. A sinner. But it didn't faze him in the least. Jesus didn't come for the people who had it all together. He came for the broken and the bleeding. For people with weepy sores like me.

After hours of dabbing my leg, I noticed something. Oh, my goodness. I'd never seen it before. But there it was—as clear as day. Right above my right knee, as obvious as the hairs standing up on my arms, I had the most distinct shiny red sore. In the perfect shape of a heart.

Jesus . . .

All my life the Lord had spoken to me in different ways, but never like this: through an ugly, weeping heart-shaped sore. And the words were simple . . .

Ema, go with your heart.

His whisper was gentle but sure—and it made sense. My heart leaped. I finally knew my answer: God wanted me to keep my leg.

When I told Dr. Otley, he stared at me blankly. "What was that?"

"The leg stays," I repeated.

Dr. William F. Marshall, one of the other five doctors from the day before, shook his head, aghast.

Good thing Dr. Otley spoke first. "Ema, did you hear what I said before? Your body's being attacked. This infection has only gotten worse. Just look at your toes. They're black and dying."

"Maybe so, but I know what I need to do."

Dr. Marshall sat himself down so his face was only a few inches away from mine. "You mean to tell me you wouldn't amputate your leg to save your life?"

"Well, if you put it that way, I guess the answer is no. And the reason is because I don't have the least bit of peace about taking it off."

Dr. Otley eyed Dr. Marshall and rubbed his forehead. "Well, I hope you give it some serious thought. Soon."

"Oh, I've given it plenty," I said. "And if the good Lord decides to take me home, we'll just have to let nature take its course. I'm in God's hands, so ... we'll just have to wait and see."

I really didn't know what would happen to me, but I'd made up my mind. I was going to take one painful day at a time.

I took that Australian doctor's suggestion to try horse chestnut extract, and wouldn't you know, it actually started to help a little.

For comfort I camped in the book of Job, and the more I did, the more I wanted to high-five the guy. And I would someday, but hopefully not for a long while. I thought of his words in Job 3:24: "For sighing has become my daily food; my groans pour out like water."

For one thing, I didn't eat daily food. And for another thing, I groaned. My groans didn't pour out like water—but my sores sure did!

This is just a test, I reminded myself. Like I kept reminding my soul who was in charge: *I'm not my own. Even my legs are not my own.*

Three months after Dr. Otley wanted to amputate my leg, the sores, infections, and blood clots all cleared up and went away. Everyone was amazed. I had only one thing to say:

Thank you, Jesus!

The sores had left a lot of scars, but I could sure handle those. Scars were nothing like sores. Scars were actually healed wounds. On Jesus, they were proofs of his faithfulness to his Father—even in the face of death. Not only that, but they were proof of his Father's faithfulness to him—right to the end.

Out of Options

As I sat on my deck watching the pink clouds roll in, I thought about my Daddy's health, which had taken a nosedive lately.

God, you know how much I want to be there for him. How much I want to take him to his doctor's appointments and help him like he helped me when Eddie left. I feel so limited ...

Ellie had known Daddy for a long time, so she could be an extension of me and take Daddy to his doctor appointments. We had a plan: Ellie would pick him up from my brother Murray's house where he lived and call me right after the appointment so I could find out how it went. It wasn't as good as being there, but it gave me a chance to be involved and help make decisions.

I appreciated Ellie doing so much, but I still felt the ache inside. I'd always wanted to help Daddy the way I'd helped Mom.

Please talk to me, Jesus. I'm listening and waiting ...

I didn't hear anything except the birds. A cardinal snatched some seed from the feeder next door while a robin hopped around in the grass, reminding me of Matthew 6:26: "Look at the birds of the air; they do not sow or reap or store away in barns, and yet your heavenly Father feeds them. Are you not much more valuable than they?"

Birds come in so many varieties, but nobody ever heard of a robin being jealous of a cardinal. It just didn't happen. Birds accepted their situations. And here I was, wrestling with pain, crookedness, and this never-ending sense of my uselessness.

Hungry for help, I riffled through the Bible to find a verse I'd read. There it was—Romans 9:20–21: "But who are you, a human being, to talk back to God? 'Shall what is formed say to the one who formed it, "Why did you make me like this?"' Does not the potter have the right to make out of the same lump of clay some pottery for special purposes and some for common use?"

I knew God didn't make me like this, but he sure allowed it. I didn't understand it, but I needed to accept it. Whether God used me for a special purpose or for some simple common use shouldn't matter. At least I didn't want it to matter. I wanted to feel privileged that he'd even use me in the first place.

It might not *feel* fair that I was too crippled to help Daddy, but it *was* fair. Because God is fair. After all, he balances everything out in the end. The last would be first and all that kind of stuff. I knew it, but somehow I had to latch on to it all over again. The little seed of trust God gave me yesterday wouldn't be enough to carry me through today.

It was just like the time in the Bible when God supplied the Israelites only enough manna for one day. The previous day's manna would always go bad. Just like the Israelites, I needed my daily portion of fresh truth. I chuckled. How funny that God could use anything in all of creation to remind me of these things. Even a little robin hopping around.

Heavenly Daddy, help me trust you about my earthly daddy. Thank you for providing Ellie, and thank you that Daddy is in good hands. Especially because he's in your hands.

As I continued to pray and stir up my faith, something came over me. Jesus slipped a bit of sweet peace into my mind: *It's going to be okay, Ema. I'm going to take care of you—and take care of your daddy too.*

June 17, 2008

As I waited in Dr. Bengston's office, I felt a sense of dread about what I needed to say. My last several appointments had felt more like disappointments. His normally smiling face had faded, and to me, he seemed a little disconnected, almost disinterested.

My heart raced because I didn't want to talk to him about my feelings. But at the same time, I didn't want to go on pretending it didn't bother me—because it did. Maybe something bothered him. Maybe it drove him crazy that he couldn't fix me. I wouldn't blame him. After all, he was the RSD expert, and all these years my RSD symptoms just kept getting worse. But to me, something didn't feel right.

I had discussed my feelings with Dr. Cindy—even about the possibility of switching doctors. She listened and understood, then suggested I talk to Dr. Bengston about it directly.

But Lord, I feel like I need another confirmation about what to do. You hear my heart. Please show me if what I'm thinking is the right thing.

A few minutes later, Dr. Bengston walked in with a faraway look in his eyes. My heart fell. Okay, here goes ...

"You probably want to know what's happening with my pain."

"Go ahead." He crossed his arms, and his eyes glazed over in sudden tiredness.

I felt the heat rise to my cheeks. I'd been working with this guy for twelve years. My stomach twisted and my mouth felt like chalk, but I had to do this, didn't I?

"Dr. Bengston? I've been thinking ..."

He cocked an eyebrow. "Oh? Go ahead. What about?"

I cleared my throat. "About us." I groaned. That wasn't the way I wanted to say it. Goodness, I sounded like a nervous teenager about to break up with her boyfriend. I drew in a breath to take another stab at it. "Dr. Bengston, I don't feel like I've been getting the kind of support I need. Whenever I come here, I feel like I'm wasting your time."

There, I'd said it. I studied his normally smiling face and tried not to be eaten by his silence.

Please, Lord, may this not hurt him.

Even as I prayed, something told me I had, and I felt crushed.

"Really? Hmm, I had no idea you felt that way. I'm really sorry."

I shrugged. "It's okay. Well, it's not okay, but you know what I mean." Boy, did I want this to be over. I tried again. "Dr. Bengston? I was wondering ... would it be possible for you to switch me to a different RSD specialist?"

He stepped back. "You want to see somebody else?"

There it was. The punch. I drew in a breath. "Yes. That's what I'd like."

I swallowed. If I'd hurt him, he did a good job hiding it — keeping so calm and everything. He probably just wanted to make the situation easier for me.

He eyed me intently. Was he thinking of talking me out of it? I hoped not, because if he did, I didn't know if I'd be strong enough.

"I see where you're going with this, Ema. And I'll see what I can do. I will say this: It might not be easy for you to switch doctors at this point. Doctors really hesitate to take on new patients who are on so many large doses of medicine. Especially patients who are on as many as you."

Unfixable

July 2008

I'd just finished gagging down my daily stash of pills when Jason came over. With sagging shoulders and a sad, tired face, he dropped into my kitchen chair.

"I just got divorce papers in the mail," he said.

"Oh, honey ..." There were no words. I'd known they were having marital struggles, but nothing could have prepared me for this. Helpless, I reached for his hand.

"She decided to live with her mom in New Mexico." His voice cracked as he said it, staring off.

Was this really happening? I pictured the young couple at the altar. Their promises still rang in my ears. And right now, from my bent-over position, Brady and Connor smiled at me from the refrigerator. Their photos began to blur as I prayed aloud ...

"Father, bring comfort. May Jason feel your arms around him. Thank you that you promise to be with him and never leave him. You are good and faithful. Thank you that Jason means everything to you. He's your precious son who you'll always care for no matter what."

My heart broke for him as he sat there quietly. I knew he'd open up with me when he was good and ready. He'd spill it all out, raw and uncensored—the same way I'd taught him and his brother to bring everything to God.

I'd felt that same slam of defeat when Eddie walked out. "I'm here for you, Jason."

174

"But the boys," he said. "I can't stop thinking about them. How are they going to take this?"

As he wiped his eyes, I didn't even try to be the strong one. Instead, I asked him for a Kleenex and entered his pain. What else could I do besides Romans 12:15? "Mourn with those who mourn."

Surely God felt it too. He wouldn't say "mourn with those who mourn" if he wasn't prepared to take his own advice and cry right along with us.

August 11, 2008

"Dr. Bengston's right," my primary physician said at our next appointment. "It won't be easy to find another doctor at this point."

What had I done? Had I cut myself off from the only RSD doctor who would even consider me? So had God given me the go-ahead or not? Had I missed something?

"Don't sweat it," Dr. Bell said, sensing my disappointment. "Dr. Bengston and I will keep trying to find someone. In the meantime, we can do more diagnostic testing. If you're up to it, that is."

"No, thank you," I said.

He nodded. "I know the testing aggravates your RSD. I certainly understand you not wanting to do it. Unfortunately, however, it's tricky to do anything at such an advanced stage. Are you still going to counseling?"

I laughed. "Oh, yeah."

"Good. Because at this point, it's probably one of the best things to help you cope." He paused. "How *is* the pain level?"

"Indescribable."

He shook his head with compassion. "Well, Dr. Bengston's doing a great job managing all your pain medication. I see he just authorized more thalidomide and morphine. Be sure to keep calling his nurse when you need more refills, okay?"

"Oh, that reminds me. I'm having the worst time taking my pills.

Every time I swallow, it burns my throat. It feels like I have a big lump in there."

He sighed. "Hmm, I think we need to set you up with your gastro-enterologist."

January 21, 2009

After years of seeing so many different doctors, I had a favorite. Dr. Amindra Arora. I liked him for a lot of reasons. Right from our first visit, this sweet little man from India with the wide animated grin showed the deepest concern for me. For example, when I told him his doorway was a bit too narrow for me, he took it very seriously. At my next visit, his nurse said she had a surprise for me. And she took me to a different room. A room they mostly used for wide equipment. There Dr. Arora had hung a sign that said, "Ema's Room." It was like a hug from heaven.

Just then, Dr. Arora walked in. I don't know what amused me more—his polka-dotted bow tie or his mismatched socks—but these were the kind of things that so endeared me to him.

His dark, happy eyes danced from behind his black-rimmed glasses. "Ema! It's good to see you!"

"Oh, it's good to see you too, Dr. Arora."

"I understand you've been having heartburn and your fluids aren't staying down. And you've been choking and aspirating." He shook his head sadly. "This doesn't sound good. We want your drinks in your stomach, not in your lungs."

Despite the topic, he made me smile. "It burns whenever I swallow, and there's a constant lump in my throat. It feels like there's a blockage."

His face wrinkled in concentration. "It sounds like we need to do an EGD. We can send a little tube down there with a camera on the end and take a look. We'll check your esophagus, stomach, and the first part of the small intestine. Of course, we'll put you to sleep first."

"Oh, that won't work," I said. "I can't take general anesthesia any-more. Unfortunately, I've developed some kind of an allergy. But go ahead. You can still do the procedure. You'll just have to keep me awake."

He raised his eyebrows. "Okay. I'll order the EGD, but I think I'll have one of my other colleagues do it."

January 23, 2009

"Now, remember," the gastroenterologist said, "it's crucial that you stay completely still."

"Don't worry, I'm not going anywhere," I assured him. With that, I opened my mouth for the tube.

How did he feel about this? Was he nervous? Goodness, I wouldn't blame him if he was. It's not every day you stick a tube down a crooked lady's throat while she stares back at you.

Don't think about what he's doing, I told myself. I have to admit, it wasn't easy. Not with his gloved hands in my face.

When I thought about hands, I willed myself to think of some-thing more pleasant — like Connor. I remembered how he'd shared some personal concerns with me about his missing fingers.

"I wish I could be like other kids," he said. "They all have normal hands."

I felt his ache. There had to be something I could do to help him see the value in his uniqueness. Later, when he excused himself to go to the bathroom, God gave me an idea. I wheeled over to my vanity and carefully removed my Franklin Mint sculpture of Jesus. I loved this delicate piece with all its details. That's why it made me cringe when I considered what I had to do.

Go for it, I told myself. It will be worth the sacrifice. So, gritting my teeth, I broke off three of Jesus' fingers.

"Hey, look," I said, when Connor got back, "Jesus is missing fin-gers, but he still looks perfect and beautiful. See? Even with fewer fingers, you can do everything God wants you to do. There's no limit when God lives inside you."

Connor then studied the fingerless Jesus. Kind of like me now studying the doctor's fingers — except Connor could smile.

As the doctor's hands hovered near my mouth, he stole a glance at the attending physician behind him. What was going on? Why didn't he stay focused? They made some kind of an exchange, and the second doctor suddenly stepped up and took over. Why did they do that? Was something wrong? Did the first guy feel uncomfortable with me staring at him?

To add to my fears, I suddenly had to cough. But I couldn't. I had to hold it back. My heart beat faster, and the next thing I knew, my airways tightened.

Lord, help.

Before I could even give them a warning, I threw up.

"Steady," the nurse said, holding me still.

Just when I thought they'd pull out the tube and we'd be done, they inserted a second tube. Maybe some kind of suction. I don't know.

"Don't worry," the doctor said. "We'll clean you up. Try to relax."

Relax? I couldn't even do that on a normal day. But I couldn't say anything. I could only let them snake down the rest of tube number one while I concentrated on my breathing. It wasn't until they retrieved both tubes that I gave myself the luxury of a painful cough.

"Find any blockages?" I asked.

The doctor shook his head. "No, I didn't. So far, so good."

Yeah right, I thought.

September 3, 2009

They were right about it being difficult to find a replacement doctor. A year and a half after Dr. Bengston and I parted ways, I was back in Dr. Bengston's office so we could give it another go.

Lord, please, may this not be too awkward.

Over the years, I had opportunities to casually talk to Dr. Bengston about God. Sometimes it would start with him asking about my attitude: "Ema, you're still smiling. How is that possible?"

That's when I'd tell him, "It's Jesus. He gives me all the strength I need."

I had to remember this today. In my weakness, God would be strong.

Dr. Bengston slipped in and closed the door. After briefly acknowledging Ellie and Cathy, he turned his full attention to me. "Welcome back."

His mouth curled into the same friendly smile. What did he think about my appearance? I leaned sideways off my wheelchair more than ever. At least on a sixty-degree angle. My skin looked blotchy and mottled — white with little reddish, bluish clusters.

"You're still smiling," he said.

I chuckled. "For the same reason as before."

He gave a knowing look. "Because of your faith."

"You got it. And today I'm smiling for another reason too."

"Oh, yeah? What's that?"

"Because I get to see you again."

"Thank you, Ema. That means a lot." He looked at his computer. "I see Dr. Bell has really increased your morphine. How is that helping your pain?"

"Not much. And right now my right hand is hurting too. I don't know what's happening. It's been stiff and sore."

"Let's take a look."

I cringed as he flexed and bent my wrist, hand, and fingers.

"I think we need to put it in a splint. I'll have the nurse give you one, and we'll have you back in a month to reevaluate."

October 7, 2009

"We do not lose heart. Though outwardly we are wasting away, yet inwardly we are being renewed day by day. For our light and momentary troubles are achieving for us an eternal glory that far outweighs them all" (2 Corinthians 4:16–17).

I meditated on Scripture as I waited for Dr. Bengston. The splint hadn't worked. I hated to tell him, but it only worsened my pain. And it took away the use of my only functioning hand. What next? Would it end up clawing too?

Jesus, thank you for your eternal glory that far outweighs all these problems. Compared to your glory, these problems are light and temporary. Thank you so much for helping me patch it up with Dr. Bengston. I don't know why I had to go through all this, but I do appreciate him, Lord. He's a good doctor. And I appreciate you too. My hands may be all messed up, but at least they're not pierced and bleeding like yours were. And my spine may be all bent to the side, but at least it isn't pinned against a cross. You endured all that for me, so the least I can do is give all my praise back to you.

"Good morning," Dr. Bengston said cheerfully. "How's the hand?"

"Not good," I said, sticking it out so he could remove the splint.

I sucked in a breath as he squeezed my hand in a few different places.

"I'm not yet sure what's going on," he said, puzzled. "We could do an electromyogram, which basically measures the electrical activity in the muscles as they rest and contract."

"More testing?" I said.

"I could skip the test and give you a steroid injection, but we don't want to stir up the RSD."

"How about we do nothing," I said. "Because nothing seems to work anyway."

I didn't say it angrily. It was simply a fact—and he knew it. That's why he dictated the following in his medical report:

> We might not find anything that is actually fixable in her case, and we are certainly limited in regards to what we can do from an intervention standpoint.

Deadly Dose

March 2010

While Brady and Connor wolfed down some milk and oatmeal cookies, Jeff and Jason tried to convince me to use the Facebook page they'd set up for me.

"Ah, come on," Jason said. "It would be a good way to keep up with everybody."

Daddy sat in his blue chair, taking us in, like his evening entertainment.

"I don't know anything about Facebook," I said, trying to think of a way to change the subject.

Jason wiped some stray crumbs from the table. "It's easy. I'll show you."

"I'll even friend you," Jeff said, giving me one of his dramatic smiles.

I gave them a look. "What is this? Peer pressure from my own kids?"

Of course, they knew I'd pray about it. I prayed about everything. If anybody could convince me of anything, the Lord could.

And that's what happened. When I prayed about it, he reminded me how I could use my words to bring encouragement to others. So it was settled. And on March 6, 2010, I wrote my first Facebook post:

What is your response when trouble arises? You can choose to accept difficulty as a blessing by letting it deepen your relationship with Christ. Whether your current circumstances are good or painful, take time to be still before the Lord.

It didn't take me long to find RSD support groups and start posting words of hope on their walls. Friend requests started trickling in, and boy, did I love my new stranger-friends. Before I knew it, I had myself quite the active community for the suffering.

One woman wrote,

Beautiful posts, Ema. You provide inspiration and quiet strength in our moments of pain and despair. You always reach out your hand to anyone suffering and remind us how blessed we are. Thank you for showing us that we are never alone and to keep our faith!

How overwhelming to know I could make a difference right from my own little office.

Thank you, Jesus, for opening the door so I could help other hurting people see they're not alone.

As the days went on, my body plummeted in a silent, invisible war. I couldn't imagine it getting any worse. I leaned sideways even more. And the more I leaned, the more I hurt. With everything in me, I hoped nobody else would ever have to experience this. I'd met a few others on Facebook with RSD, but I doubted anyone else had become so twisted, so bent and deformed. I often felt alone.

I reread passages like Philippians 4:5 – 7: "Let your gentleness be evident to all. The Lord is near. Do not be anxious about anything, but in every situation, by prayer and petition, with thanksgiving, present your requests to God. And the peace of God, which transcends all understanding, will guard your hearts and your minds in Christ Jesus."

Okay, Father, I need your peace that transcends understanding. I lean into you. Please help this pain to go away. Please show me what to do — if anything.

September 13, 2010

Just to throw another monkey wrench in things, at the height of my pain, insurance stopped paying for my thalidomide. Probably because it cost a ton more than the morphine.

Dr. Bell shook his head as he stared at the insurance letter, probably trying to find the words.

"What are we going to do?" I asked.

He blew out a slow, even breath. "How's the pain level?"

"Off the charts. I really couldn't imagine it getting any worse." And it was true. The pain was constant and inescapable. It stalked me wherever I went. Even the smallest things could set it off: someone switching on a lightbulb, a semitruck rumbling by in the distance ... Anything and everything could ignite my abnormal nerve endings. Something as small as a breeze could cause electrical impulses to fire at Mach force. Boy, if only I could unplug it and short-circuit the process.

Dr. Bell looked at his computer. "You're taking 800 milligrams of morphine and 400 mg of thalidomide. The thalidomide has been really helping your pain. So if we need to get you off it, we'll have to raise your morphine."

I tried to swallow. "What do you want to raise it to? I can't imagine the dose getting any higher."

"I know," he said, sighing. "It's kind of an extra big jump this time."

My throat felt dry. "How big?"

"I'd like to increase it to 1600 milligrams."

"You're right," I said. "That *is* an extra big jump."

"I know. But we need to make up for the loss of the thalidomide. You're already at an extremely high pain level, so it's the best thing we can do." His eyes returned to the insurance letter. "Since they won't pay for your thalidomide after October 4, we want to boost your morphine to 1600 milligrams over these next two weeks. Of course, we'll have to keep a close eye on you."

Did he really say 1600 milligrams? My voice felt weak as the words dragged out slow. "Have you ever given that much morphine to anybody else?"

He quickly shook his head. "No, but at this point, Ema, we're just trying to keep you comfortable."

Keep me comfortable? Wasn't that something they did for dying people? Is that what we'd come to?

I knew what this drug could do to me. Every morphine jump had been brutal, and every time my body tried to fight and resist it. The cruel reality of his words sank in. The doctors had exhausted all possibilities. They simply didn't know what to do with me anymore.

As soon as I got home, I called Jason at work. "You won't believe this. Dr. Bell increased my morphine from 800 milligrams to 1600. The jump's going to happen over these next two weeks."

"He did what?"

"They're moving me up to 1600 milligrams of morphine," I repeated. "That's sixteen pills a day—not even counting all my other medications."

"That's ridiculous ... 1600 milligrams? I don't know about that."

I heard the worry in his voice, but for once I didn't know how to encourage him.

The brutal side effects kicked in faster and stronger than any of us expected. Pain gripped me from the inside out, ripping into me with more gagging and vomiting than I'd ever known. My heart raced so fast I could hardly tell the beats apart. My whole townhome blurred around me. I slurred my speech and forgot things.

"Cathy, did I drink my Boost?"

"I gave it to you after we fed the cats, remember?"

My mind felt like mush. I shook and trembled, which only further traumatized my spine. My mood went up and down like a yo-yo. I couldn't do much except hang off my wheelchair, shaking, gagging, and struggling for breath. I threw myself at Jesus' feet like never before.

I'm broken, Jesus. Crumbled to pieces. Please carry me ...

He knew every mumble-jumbled thought and he stayed close. Closer than ever.

You're with me even when I can't hear you—I know you are. You feel each stinging tear, and you collect them in your bottle, don't you, God? Please remind me you do ...

Dr. Bell and Dr. Cindy called to check on me several times a day—to make sure I was still alive. But mostly I couldn't talk to them. I could only groan and make noises.

Dr. Cindy assured me she was praying for me. "If anybody can get through this, it's my Ema. I know you can."

"Hang in there," Dr. Bell said. "We've given you a monster dose. It takes time for the body to adjust."

Cathy and Ellie were nearly beside themselves. They'd seen me face a dozen giants, but never anything like this. Helpless, I hung off my chair like a wet dishrag. I couldn't even string sentences to calm the fear in their faces.

I hated this morphine increase—but what could I do? With the thalidomide on its way out of my system, the pain would be unbearable without it.

This desert I'd been thrown into was much more dangerous than the others, but Jesus would see me through. He always had. I had no reason to doubt him now.

Jesus, I remember how you put your hand on my shoulder and pulled me out of that pit of despair. Please place your hand on me again. You

spoke and commanded life when I couldn't breathe. Revive me again. And
be my oasis.

Cathy, Ellie, and other close friends wrote on my Facebook page, asking people for serious prayer for me. Supportive emails and messages
poured in, but as the days turned into weeks, we still didn't know if
I'd make it.

One of my friends wrote on my wall:

> It has been one month of suffering this horrific pain for Ema!
> Our hearts are moved daily as we see her reach for God with
> this incredible strength and hope. She refuses to be discouraged
> because she deeply believes that God will do what he says. And
> she knows God's plan will continue on God's schedule!
>
> He continues to bless her with a clear and strong mind,
> despite the alarming amounts of medication. Ema daily thanks
> God for his goodness and grace. We all find joy in knowing
> that Ema lives within God's constant care! Thank you all for
> being such loyal friends through this very difficult time! What
> sweet comfort to know that what we do for others, we do for
> God. Blessings to all!

Moving On

December 2010

After three long, horrific months of suffering, my body finally started to tolerate this crazy new level of morphine. I'd made it to the other side, and I was still alive—*thank you, Jesus!*

You'd think such an insane amount of morphine would take a good slice out of my pain, but with the thalidomide out of my system, the pain only escalated. I felt trapped. Stuck in my own body.

And something else bothered me too. Over the years, I'd seen handicapped people withdraw and become prisoners in their own homes. The last thing I wanted was to become a recluse. It could happen so easily, especially with *my* mountain of challenges. What a terrifying thought. But this wasn't for me. No matter what, I couldn't lose touch with the outside world.

"We need to get me out," I said.

"Tell us where you'd like to go," Cathy said, "and we'll try to make it happen."

"Well, for starters, you could take me shopping again."

Shopping was no small deal, and they knew it—because of what it involved to get me ready. After all, I had my dignity. Instead of my usual sponge bath, I'd need to clean up in the shower. But with RSD, that was like subjecting me to the torture chamber.

Cathy got into her shorts and tank top, then opened the accordion shower curtain for me. To make it easier to wash my hair, she backed me in. Of course, my wheelchair stuck out, so they had to throw towels on the floor.

"Here comes the facecloth," Ellie said. My teeth clenched down, diverting the pain, but it didn't erase it.

"I'll try to make this as quick as possible," Cathy said. I braced myself as she picked up the showerhead. As she cranked the handle, my breathing broke into a series of fitful gusts and starts. Left and right, water knifed into my skin.

She set down the sprayer. "Here comes the shampoo. Hang in there just a few more seconds." But every second felt like a minute and every minute like an hour. Each water droplet stabbed my bare skin.

Keep the vision, I told myself. You're having this shower because you want to be with the girls at Walmart. You want to feel useful. You want to be able to smile, connect with people, and feel somewhat human again.

The water made its last few heavy jabs, but I knew better than to feel too relieved — because next came the towels. Unfortunately, even the gentlest blots gave new meaning to the phrase "getting on my nerves."

Cathy and Ellie knew I needed time to recover after my shower, so they draped towels over me and wheeled me to my bedroom. There I'd wait it out for half an hour before we wrestled me into my clothes.

As the tears fell, I tried to talk truth to my soul. Tried to cancel Satan's lies and shift my focus from my situation to my destination. God didn't just keep me alive so I could take up space. He had a purpose for me.

From under the towels, I thought about Luke 11:33: "No one lights a lamp and puts it in a place where it will be hidden, or under a bowl. Instead they put it on its stand, so that those who come in may see the light."

You're my destination, Jesus!

I also thought about the apostle Paul, one of the brightest lights in the New Testament. As a religious zealot, he hated Christians so much he wanted them dead. He would even try to trick them so he could arrest them for blasphemy and drag them off to prison. And that was exactly what he planned to do in Damascus before the risen Jesus appeared to him in a rush of bright light.

Hearing Jesus' voice, Paul fell to the ground and cried, "Who are you?"

The Lord replied, "I am Jesus, whom you are persecuting."

God, in his goodness, saw Paul's spiritual blindness and struck him blind temporarily. He made him blind physically so he could open Paul's eyes spiritually and lead him to the true lasting light. From a place of affliction, God called Paul to restore others and bring them to that same lasting light.

That's what I want to do, Lord Jesus. Bring others to your light.

"Okay, I'm ready!" I hollered to Cathy and Ellie.

We started with my bottom half first. After we worked my pants to my ankles, I used my right arm to slowly inch myself up. Such tiny movements were excruciating. I had to press my left torso into my left arm. While I pushed, they pulled. It took several painful tries to get it right. And when we finally did, we still had my upper clothing to deal with. The whole process from undressing to showering and redressing took more than three hours. And then we still had the drive ahead of us.

Bill had become a master at angling me into the R&S van, but I still held my breath until I got safely inside.

"How are the kids?" I asked as he fastened me in. After all these years of driving with him, I felt as if I'd watched them grow up.

"They ask about you," he said, putting the van in gear.

"Really? Did you tell them about my latest morphine increase?"

"I sure did, and we're relieved you made it through."

Minutes later, I broke into chills and sweats. Not again, I thought.

In addition to my ongoing breathing problems, I also had to deal with this temperature problem. Like edema and joint problems, the chills snuck up and threw me into their game of unpredictability.

You like to keep life interesting, don't you, Lord? Well, could you please keep me calm so I can get to the store in one piece? No broken ribs or anything, okay?

Everything went fine for the first ten minutes. Then the tremors started. Pain rattled me inside and out, jolting my stomach. Cathy didn't have to ask. She knew.

"Here you go," she said, handing me the bucket. I stepped into the routine so naturally that after we cleaned me up, I jumped right back into conversation. Such was my way in this predictably unpredictable life.

From my lopsided angle, I saw the tall smattering of streetlamps and knew we'd reached the Walmart parking lot.

Bill wheeled me down the ramp, and I smiled at an employee pushing a bunch of carts. One time an employee lost control of his carts and they banged into my wheelchair. Talk about traumatizing my spine. And who could forget the time at the bank when the automatic doors malfunctioned and closed on me. Not only did they set off my panic buttons, they set off the clerks' too.

And oh, how I hated my automatic reactions to fear. They hit me like dominos, triggering my breathing issues.

I took a deep breath as Cathy pushed me through Walmart's automatic doors. "Let the fun begin," I said. Truth was, shopping could be downright hazardous. The slightest brush of someone's arm could cause a hurricane reaction, which was why I needed both Ellie and Cathy to accompany me.

With my dangling head sticking out right in the middle of the aisle, it took two people to keep constant vigil. While Ellie pushed my wheelchair, Cathy became my human shield, protecting my head with her body and shopping cart. Together, the two of them intercepted passing carts, swinging hands, and any other surprises.

People eyed us with curiosity and concern. Let's face it. I was a head turner. My head hung at about the same level as the average person's belly button and backside, depending on what way they were standing. So if we weren't careful, we could get ourselves into all kinds of trouble. A few months before, I had a bad experience on an elevator. A woman carrying a portable potty, of all things, ignored Cathy's warning that there wasn't room. She stared at me like I should sit up or something—as if I could. Then she forced her way in and stood right in front of my head. My eyeballs were literally six inches away from her toilet lid!

Thank goodness Walmart didn't have elevators—just people. After a few minutes in the store, a concerned lady stepped over.

"I'm a nurse. Can I help her sit up?"

This never got easier. "No, thanks," Cathy said. "Ema can't sit up."

I didn't have the energy to worry about it. Instead, I looked at our grocery list. We needed vegetable broth, milk, orange juice, peach juice, vanilla ice cream, bottled water, chicken nuggets for Brady and Connor's visits, Lysol cleaning spray, sponges, a new hair brush, and a bag of cat food.

Most people walked the aisle only once, but my only way to see both sides was to have the girls take me down twice—once on the left side and once on the right. On the bright side, though, it sometimes gave me a second chance to connect with people.

"How's it going?" I asked a little girl looking in my direction.

She glanced at her mother. "Fine, thanks."

I caught her whisper, "It's the crooked lady." But the phrase didn't bother me. People were just stating the facts. I was crooked. That was just a fact of life.

Cathy and Ellie moved like pros. What a blessing. I made a point of thanking them regularly. Frankly, I couldn't imagine life without them, and I didn't expect I'd need to.

September 2011

Ellie leaned her broom against the kitchen counter. "My fibromyalgia hasn't been cooperating. I don't know how else to say this, but I think it's time to retire."

My mind skittered in a dozen different directions. Retire? No—she couldn't do that. I needed her too much. Ellie was more than a caregiver. She was a friend. That's what she'd been to me from the beginning. Losing her would practically be like losing an arm and a leg. I couldn't tell her that though. Not now. Instead I told her, "You need to do what you think is best." And I knew what to do after we said good night. I retreated to my secret place.

Father! What now? With my health going down, I need Ellie more than ever. Who could possibly replace her?

The Lord knew the job qualities I wanted in a caregiver. She had to be trustworthy, caring, intelligent, conscientious, clean, precise, teachable, fun, funny, and, of course, detailed—just to name a few. Oh, and I also wanted someone who would get along with Cathy. *So tell me, God. Who could possibly fit all these things?*

Just then, Jason popped up in my mind. What in the world? I must have been overtired or something. Whoever heard of someone's son becoming her caregiver?

I rolled myself into my office to think more about this. Jason was facing uncertainties with his job and wanted more security—so why *not* Jason? When it came right down to it, he fit all my job qualifications.

When he phoned later that week, we talked about Connor and Brady and different things like that. Then, out of the blue, the Holy Spirit whispered, *Ask him now.*

I swallowed. "Ah, Jason? What would you think about becoming my caregiver?"

He cleared his throat. "Well, I hadn't really thought about it."

"Well, please do, because I think you'd be great. You already know most of what it involves. You'd be cleaning, vacuuming, giving me my medications, taking me to doctor appointments. Doing just about everything except the real personal stuff."

Two and a half days later, he got back to me. "I'll do it."

"Really?" My heart warmed at God's great provision.

Thank you, Jesus. You're truly my number one caregiver.

Preparation

December 23, 2011

Christmas choruses filled the air as Cathy and I worked in the kitchen. She set down a bowl of well-beaten liquids on the chair in front of me. Then, after pouring in the flour, baking soda, and salt, she handed me a mixing spoon.

"Stir away," she said, keeping her hand on the bowl. How many times had we done this over the years? I'd lost count, but it never got old.

She poured in the chocolate chips, and I set down my spoon. "Got something for you." Before she could blink, I smeared a speck of batter on her hand.

"Hey! Two can play at that game." And with that, she got me back. How we got anything done was a mystery.

"Oh, smell that ham," I said. "Jason's going to be in hog heaven." I smelled the sloppy joes too in the other slow cooker. Boy, did everything smell heavenly.

Before Cathy left at the end of the day, we'd stick the meat in the fridge with everything else: the cheese tray, salads, sweet corn, veggie tray, red and green Jell-O, and pumpkin pie. All week long, I'd been crossing off things from my list. Everything had to be ready in advance so on Christmas Eve day, I wouldn't have to do anything except call a friend to reheat things.

Cathy set the cookie sheet in front of me, and I spooned out big clumps of batter, equally spaced apart.

"You're such a perfectionist," she said.

Of course, I didn't deny it. A bit later, when someone knocked on the kitchen door, we knew who it was. We'd left the side door to the garage unlocked for Jason.

"He's back with your sweet rolls," Cathy said, wiping her hands on her apron.

"Don't let him in," I reminded her. "Not until tomorrow."

Cathy slipped into the garage to retrieve the groceries.

"Thanks, honey!" I hollered.

Over the last three months, Jason had proved to be the perfect caregiver. He exceeded my expectations, and that said a lot. He and Cathy hit it off like brother and sister, just like I wanted. Their teasing and joking always added the right touch of fun.

I looked at Cathy. "Here goes the last scoop of batter, then you can stick 'em in the oven."

Not a year went by that I didn't get excited about surprising the boys with my new theme and arrangement of decorations. I couldn't wait to show them my candles, figurines, angels, lighted garlands, sparkly gift boxes, bows, and yes, even my helium balloons.

After Cathy and I finished cleaning our mess, we set the table. While shopping, I'd found the cutest porcelain "Happy Birthday, Jesus" plates.

"You know what?" I said. "We still need to set out my pine candles. What do you think?"

"I think you're going to have the most festive place in town."

"That's right. We want Jesus to feel welcome on his birthday."

After several more hours of work, we got everything exactly the way I wanted it.

"Thanks for your help," I told Cathy around midnight.

She followed me out to the deck. "Enjoy your time with Jesus."

"I will. See you on Christmas morning."

"You bet. Call me tomorrow if you need anything."

"Oh, I'll be fine," I assured her. "Enjoy your family." The door closed behind her, and I looked at the stars, shining extra bright and beautiful.

They're just like you, Jesus. You're the star of my Christmas.

It always helped to focus on him, but boy, was I tired. And I won't even get into my pain. Yup, this old girl had done it again. I'd pushed myself too hard, and now I felt it in my arms, neck, and spine. Goodness, I thought, I'm too young to feel so old. I laughed at myself.

I didn't regret all my work. How could I when I had all these fun decorations, gifts, and goodies to show for it? Besides, when I saw the wonder on everybody's faces on Christmas Eve, it would be worth it.

The Miracle

December 24, 2011, 12:15 a.m.

When the wind picked up, I knew it was time to leave the deck. Grabbing my wheel with my working hand, I used my good foot to drag forward.

You can do it, baby.

I worked my way to the door and cranked it open, but my wheels got stuck on the threshold. Groaning, I tried again.

It's worth the independence, I told myself.

One last tug and I broke loose into the kitchen, smack into the smell of sloppy joes and ham. Breathing it in, I looked at my fancy table with its place mats, plates, and goblets, and fresh excitement bubbled inside me. In nineteen hours, the boys would knock on my door and our Christmas Eve celebration would begin.

My body felt extra heavy as I pulled myself to the living room to catch my breath. Resting beneath my lighted archway, I stared at the Christmas tree with its gift-box ornaments and twinkling lights.

This birthday theme is for you, Jesus. You're our honored guest.

Closing my eyes, I rehashed my plans for the boys and smiled at my sneaky ways. This would be one Christmas we'd never forget.

I drank in a deep breath and worked my way down the hall into my office. Savannah welcomed me with a meow.

"Cheery in here, isn't it, girl?"

I glanced at the dolls on the shelves. Such sweet gifts from my sons. Even now, they kept the memories alive.

It felt good to park under my desk and turn on my computer. I might be a tough old bird, but at least I could still encourage others on Facebook.

I scrolled to my latest post. December 17, 2011:

Matthew 1:23: "The virgin will conceive and give birth to a son, and they will call him Immanuel (which means 'God with us')." In the midst of this wonderful Christmas season, my friends, we must all remember that God is always with us wherever we are. Blessings to you!

What a promise. Immanuel ... God with us.

Lord Jesus, may everyone who reads this post find lasting hope in you.

I prayed about what to write, and a verse from Matthew popped into my head: "With God all things are possible." Good one, but where was the reference? Scanning my room sideways, I spotted my Bible on my second desk. I'd have to back up to grab it, but no big deal. I did it all the time.

Reaching for my wheel, I pushed off with my right foot while turning. But I must not have pulled back far enough because my wheelchair caught on the side of my desk. I gave it another quick push — this time with more strength — and my right wheel came off the floor ...

No —!

My heart leaped as my body flew.

Pain exploded when the curve of my neck slammed the floor, crushing it against the bend. Fire shot through my spine.

My crooked foot got pinned somewhere behind my right leg, and my left arm lay trapped beneath me. All I could see of it was my big club fist, looking lifeless and useless in front of my face.

Fear gripped me. I couldn't move. Couldn't straighten my left leg. The slightest attempt only spiked the pain. My phone sat on my desk, but I couldn't reach it.

"Help!" But it was no use. My neighbors in the townhome beside me were away for Christmas. My heart sank. Only one person could hear my gut-wrenching cries.

Jesus!

Surely he'd rescue me.

Savannah kept sticking her whiskery head in my face and leaving the room howling. I'd never heard such a desperate cry from a cat.

Jesus, is this how you're going to take me home?

I tried to focus on heaven, but sickness bit into me. I thought I'd experienced every level of pain, but I was wrong. So wrong.

Jesus, where are you? My helper, my Savior, my lifeline.

The words got stuck and I could only keep screaming his name.

"Jesus!"

I imagined him taking those nails. Yielding to blow after blow. Every time I called him, I knew he heard me. He had to. He'd listened to me all my life, even when nobody else did. Time after time, he'd rescued me. He'd never stopped caring. Even now, in my darkest hour, he wouldn't let me down. I couldn't imagine it.

The clock on my desk seemed to mock me. Thoughts of loved ones came and left. Who would find me? Who would call 911?

Hour sank into endless hour, and the pain raged on. Trapped by my own body, I could only keep screaming his name. Over and over, I screamed it, from my raw, parched throat.

"Jesus!"

Eight and a half hours passed and I was still fully awake.

Jesus, is this what it feels like to die?

Suddenly, without warning, something began to change. Something began to shift in the atmosphere.

Out of nowhere, I heard it — loud and reverberating, roaring and growing like the wind. My heart raced.

Distant and close at the same time, it consumed my whole house, closing in on me.

A powerful presence. Like I wasn't alone.

What in the world?

I held my breath as time froze. My room lit up in a sudden shock of brightness.

A tall man in a flowing white robe stood in the corner. His clothes looked alive and they glowed as they flowed, saturating him in warm, magnetic radiance. His face shone like a ball of light, and his robe was so bright, I had to keep looking away.

I struggled to believe what I saw. It felt surreal. Like I'd passed through a veil into another dimension. All my senses were heightened. An invisible language passed between us. Without doubt, I knew who this was.

Jesus.

Jesus was in my room. In *my* room. The one I'd been calling to, endlessly screaming for, had come to me. When no one else was around, he stepped in to rescue me!

I felt so powerfully drawn to him. Drawn to his rich, magnetic love. It went right through me. Swelled into the deepest part of me.

I kept trying to look at him, but he was just too bright. I shook from shock, but hope washed over me and held me tight. The One who had always been there in the past had not forgotten me. My eyes quickly returned to the fullness of his shoulders, then moved down. His hands were so big and bright as they extended from his long white sleeves. I'd never seen such big hands.

Yes, I believed this was happening, but I'd never heard of Jesus visiting anybody before. My heart drummed in my chest, but everything about him only pulled me closer.

Jesus.

From the floor, he looked like he almost reached the ceiling. The radiant layers of his robe tousled around him, soft and breeze-like.

He stood only two or three feet away from my crumpled, pain-gripped body. He didn't touch me, and I didn't try to touch him. I didn't need to. His power swept in and through me.

Peace.

I felt the warm, gentle weight of his presence, invigorating and alive, washing over my body. Jesus stayed in front of me, but I also felt him inside of me. His rich heat moved in and through my crooked left foot, permeating it.

What happened next totally overwhelmed me. Jesus didn't physically touch me—his hands stayed open at his sides—but my crooked foot, still pinned beneath me, began to straighten. My bones cracked as my foot and leg shifted. In that moment, Jesus healed my foot and it felt completely different.

I drew in a breath. My *hand* now ...

As I felt the heat, the fingers of my closed club fist began to open on their own—slowly—but they were opening.

If I'd ever wondered what my hand would look like if it were to be opened after all these years, I didn't need to wonder anymore. Through streams of my tears, I saw it: *My open hand. All of it. Its blood-cracked lines, big open sores, and red raw flesh.*

I hardly had time to process it, because in the next second, starting with my palm and moving in the direction of my fingers, Jesus caused my hand to grow brand-new flesh. Right in front of my eyes, he covered and re-created fresh new skin over that raw, exposed hand. Over my palm and each of my fingers.

There were no words. I simply stared, shook, and sobbed. For the first time in all these years, I was flexing my fingers. Me—controlling my own hand!

The same powerful current that coursed through my foot and hand now began to straighten my neck. If the other bones cracked loud, that was nothing compared to the sound in my ears. But let the bones crack. I didn't care. Because Jesus was here. And that same healing heat now made its way from the top of my neck to the bottom of my spine. *His power ... flowing ... growing ...* Jesus was straightening my body!

The next thing I knew, I was on my back. Had Jesus put me there? He must have because I didn't remember rolling over. I didn't think I could. I melted into the floor, smitten. All his. Jesus had fixed my hand, my foot, and now my neck and spine. He'd loved me from head to toe. Trusted me with the biggest miracle I'd ever heard of.

Then, like a gentleman, he got down on one knee. Jesus got down on one knee and held out his hand to me. His right hand.

"Ema, give me your hand."

His voice … it rolled over me and through me like a thousand rushing waters. I'd heard this voice before in the hospital say, "Ema, breathe!" But this time he wasn't commanding. Only inviting.

As he stood over me, I had only one response: complete trust. Abandon. I'd do whatever he said. I'd trust him with everything in me. Like the rest of my body, my hand shook as I raised it. I was now lifting my newly reconstructed hand. Time stopped as we touched. *Waves of warmth. Strength I'd never known.* My heart was completely taken over. Lost in him.

My palm was now in the palm of Jesus Christ!

He reached for my other hand.

Rivers passed between us as his hands clasped over mine.

What was this? This sinking and soaring all at the same time …

Everything felt right about touching him, holding on to him. This was the One I was made for. In that suspended moment, years of hurt slipped away. If I could have stayed like this forever, I would have, but Jesus had something else in mind. Without a word, he brought me to my feet.

When I say "brought me to my feet," I don't mean he pulled or tugged; I mean he moved the two of us to a standing position. We rose together. In seconds, he floated us up. After all those years in my wheelchair, *I was standing on my own two feet. On my own two legs.*

My muscles didn't have a clue what to do. I wobbled as I stood. Wobbled and shook. But Jesus didn't grip me any tighter. He gave me a few seconds to let it sink in, then he let go of my hands. Oh, man. I knew what he wanted me to do. He wanted me to *walk*.

The very thought of it would have normally scared me to death, but if Jesus wanted me to walk, I could do this. After all, he was with me.

Help me, Jesus.

I put one shaky foot in front of the other, and like a toddler, I staggered out of my office, one drunken-like step at a time. I held the wall, but *I was walking*. I was carrying myself straight down the hall with Jesus right behind me. One step, then another. My body still hurt, but I kept moving forward.

I was about to keep going, but when we reached my bedroom, Jesus put his hand on my shoulder and gently turned me. Directed me to go inside.

Jesus stepped behind me as I walked into my bedroom.

He led me to my bed. And without effort, my body turned and lowered into a sitting position. I hadn't sat on my bed for *years*. Not even since I'd moved to this house. I'd used it only for guests.

Jesus stayed by my bed, glowing in that bright white robe I could hardly look at. He didn't touch me from the outside. He didn't need to, but I felt his power lifting my feet off the floor and setting my legs on the bed.

My body felt hugged by my mattress, just like I felt hugged by Jesus. Breathing deep, I reached up with my brand-new left hand and adjusted one of the pillows behind my head. I soaked in the feel of that pillow. Soaked in Jesus, joy, and hope, all in a spill of tears and laughter.

I don't know how long I stayed there. Half an hour, forty-five minutes, maybe an hour. But then Jesus lifted me back to a sitting position. He did it the same way he lowered my body onto the bed. He just did it, and there I was, sitting up.

Jesus stood me back to my feet, and that's when things changed.

I took a few steps, and as fast as he showed up, he was gone. The bright robe disappeared. So did the wind-like roar. I now moved my body on my own. Jesus wasn't moving it. I knew he was with me in the sense that he'd always been with me, but that warm electric feeling inside my body had faded away.

Under normal circumstances, this would have upset me, but it didn't because Jesus had just given me a miracle—my foot, my hand, my neck, my spine. He'd straightened everything out!

I felt like a little kid on Christmas trying out new toys, except my new toys were body parts. Holding the wall, I staggered to the bathroom and bent low to run water from the faucet. *My fingers worked.* I looked in the mirror and studied myself this way and that. I liked my new posture. Talk about improvement. I looked completely different. How fun to see all of me standing straight in full height. I stumbled through the house, opening and closing doors and drawers, loving every minute.

Thank you, Jesus. I said it over and over, knowing he heard me— just like he always heard me.

Thank you, Jesus, and a million thank yous!

Christmas Eve

December 24, 2011, 8:00 p.m.

Holding furniture for support, I tripped through the kitchen and living room, laughing and lighting candles. The boys usually took care of this when they arrived, but why wait for them when I could do it myself? I laughed. How could it be that just hours before I lay contorted on the floor, screaming Jesus' name like there was no tomorrow, and now I couldn't stop giggling like a schoolgirl.

The boys would arrive any minute, and I still needed a plan to reveal the new me.

God, can you help me? This miracle, this awesome healing encounter, is going to stay with them forever. They'll tell their children and their grandchildren how I saw you, how you touched me—everything.

I waited for a plan to pop in my head, but I didn't get one until I heard the doorbell. The boys always rang it before going into the garage—to let me know they'd arrived.

With no time to spare, I pushed my wheelchair to the kitchen. I then opened the door a crack, reached around the corner, and pushed the garage door button. I closed the kitchen door before anybody could see me and headed for my bedroom as fast as my wobbly legs could take me.

As I hid in my room, I heard Connor. "Isn't that Grandma's wheelchair?"

I slowly kicked out one foot in front of the other and made my way down the hall toward the kitchen. Like a bride about to meet her groom. This was my moment.

Jason looked up and then looked again, frozen. Everybody's mouth dropped open, their faces a mess of questions.

"Are you serious?" Jason said.

Ignoring my tears and drumming heart, I continued down the hall as they stared at me like they'd seen a ghost. Next to seeing Jesus in my office, this had to be my happiest moment.

Jason snapped awake and took a few steps closer. "Mom?"

"Come here," I said, opening my arms to him. For the first time in years, I gathered him into a full frontal squeeze. We shook, laughed, and blubbered all at once.

Jeff, white-faced, managed to set down his stack of gifts.

"Your turn, Jeff." And I threw my arms around my baby, absorbing the whole feel of him. I would have kept holding him except for something else.

My grandsons ... I felt a fresh wave of passion. For years I'd ached to hold them the precise way a grandmother should. For years I'd been stuck between this fierce desire and what I could actually do. And here I was, standing upright, just a few feet away—more eager to hold them than ever.

Connor clamped me into a bear hug. He felt as warm as sunshine. When I drew back to search his face, I saw bewilderment and confusion. I saw it in Brady too.

"Talk to Grandma," I said.

Brady shook his head. "Grandma, I'm kinda freaking out right now."

I scooped this tall, lean fifteen-year-old into my arms and held him close. "It's okay, honey. I think we're all freaking out right now."

We took turns exchanging hugs. When I got to Jeff a second time, he hugged me with one arm and pulled out his cell phone with the other.

I gave him a questioning look, but he'd already pressed the buttons. "Hello, Pastor Dennis? You know how we've been praying for my mom? Well, she's been healed. No, you don't get it. She's out of her wheelchair. Yeah, she's walking! She had a miracle. Yes, she's right here." He stuck the phone in my face. "Tell him."

I leaned into the phone. "It's true. I'm walking. Jesus healed me."

After the call, my mind was swirling like a whirlwind. I glanced at the table with all the food I'd set out by myself. I hadn't even needed to call anybody to help me. Brady looked stunned, so I draped an arm over his shoulder. "Why don't we all sit down?"

Jeff and Jason brought the rest of the food to the table, but they were mostly hungry for answers. How? When? Who? Where? The questions kept coming, and boy, did I love their faces when I told them the part about Jesus. When I described his robe ... his touch ... his voice. They wanted to hear every last detail.

Jeff looked mesmerized. "You mean he actually asked you to put your hand in his?"

"Yes, and it felt amazing." This floored everybody—the amazing reality of me coming into actual contact with Jesus. Touching him skin to skin. And talking about it only brought me right back, tripping me up all over again.

"What did Jesus feel like?" Connor asked.

I took a deep breath as if smelling a flower. "It felt like absolute perfect love. Like the most amazing presence I've ever felt in my life. Oh, sweetie, it's hard to put in words."

Who was I to tell them so much but so little? I almost felt like I needed to apologize. If only I could find all the right words and walk them through what had just happened. Take them back to the room so they could experience everything I'd seen and felt. It would change them forever.

Connor's eyes shone with innocence. "Grandma, can I see your hand again?" Slowly he reached for me with those little bits of a hand

I'd so grown to love. He cradled my fingers for a moment. Then he reached for my other hand so he could hold them together and make a comparison.

"This is all new skin," he said. "Smooth."

Everybody liked to feel it, to trace the lines. I laughed. I'd been doing the same thing ever since my miracle — moving my hands together, feeling the softness of my new flat flesh. A fresh habit, I guessed.

I pressed my feet together under the table and felt the straightness. I'd never get tired of this. One foot was as normal as the other. For the fun of it, I rotated my neck and leaned my body side to side.

Connor looked at me. "Are you still hurting, Grandma?"

His question threw me off guard. That was the only part I hadn't wanted to think about or admit to myself.

"Yes, I am, honey. Just not nearly as much as before. I still feel RSD in my hands and feet, but with my neck and spine all straight, my muscles and everything else feels so much better. The pain's many times more manageable."

Connor looked puzzled. "You mean you still have RSD? Why didn't God take it away like he healed everything else?"

I squeezed his hand. "That's a good question, honey. And I really don't know the answer, but I'm still praying that God will heal me. I truly believe God wouldn't have left the RSD unless he had a really good reason."

This seemed to settle it for him — the fact that God wasn't finished with me yet. Just as fast as he asked the question, everybody slipped back into being amazed by my miracle. Back to enjoying their new face-up grandma.

Jason eyed the boys. "What happened in this house is the biggest modern-day miracle I've ever heard of. Can you imagine what you would feel like if Jesus came into *your* room?"

The loud roaring wind swept back into my memory. I closed my eyes and tried to hold on to it. I never wanted to forget the sound or the majestic sight of Jesus. That flowing white bright robe. That magnetic pull of his love. One hint of the memory and I was right back there, trying to pull in everybody else along with me.

The guys got so caught up in my miracle that they hardly touched the ham, sloppy joes, potatoes, and salads. Almost everything on their "Happy Birthday, Jesus" plates got cold.

"Let's move into the living room," Jason said.

I hadn't sat in that blue plush chair for years, but here was my chance. "Jason ... give me a hand?" He steadied me as my body sank into it, feeling absolutely hugged. "It's like a touch of heaven," I said. "Well, maybe not. Jesus touching me — now *that* was a touch of heaven. Talk about a rush."

I couldn't stop talking about it. In the last eighteen and a half years, I'd been shaken by many things, but what did I really know about being shaken? All I knew was there couldn't be a better kind of shaking.

Jeff and Jason looked like they were on an adrenaline overload. As a family, we shared something so huge. Something so amazing and bonding — I doubted any of us felt worthy of it.

"Jesus, thank you for my miracle," I prayed aloud. *"We're completely humbled and overwhelmed with what you've done for us. You were here in this house. Thank you for meeting with us tonight. Even now, please speak to us as we read your beautiful Christmas story. Thank you for Brady, Connor, Jason, and Jeff and for all the great plans you have for them."*

"And thank you for Grandma," Connor said.

Jason handed me a Kleenex.

"Jesus, please teach us what you want us to learn," I continued. *"We want to help hurting people wherever we go. And happy birthday, Jesus."*

As Connor read the Christmas story from Luke 2, it took on a whole new meaning: an unlikely woman, her willingness to receive, her battle with pain and hardship, and finally, everybody's miracle of new life. Immanuel, God with us.

My grandsons savored each word as if sipping a tall steamy cup of hot apple cider. I'd never felt so close to them. Man, I loved those two.

"Okay," I said. "Let's open our gifts."

As Connor and Brady handed out presents like they'd done so many times, I thought about my original Christmas Eve plan: the singing, phone calls, and following my clues. Somehow none of that mattered anymore. God had come up with a whole new plan to make this Christmas memorable. And none of my homemade dreams or surprises could have compared.

"Oh, my goodness," I said. "How are we going to tell Cathy? She's supposed to take me to the Salvation Army tomorrow."

Jason shrugged. "We'll figure something out."

"Aren't you forgetting something?" Connor said. He gave us a look like it should be obvious. "When do we get to go to the office?"

My heart beat faster. I'd been hesitating because it almost felt like I should section it off with rope or something. I knew it was just an ordinary room, but it felt somewhat sacred now. Almost like holy ground, an off-limits sanctuary that should be left exactly the way it was when he appeared. On the other hand, I wanted to share it with my sons and grandsons.

"Okay," I said. "Let's do it. Let's at least retrace my steps." So slowly and quietly, they followed me down the hall.

I hesitated at the doorway and took a deep breath. "How about we just peek inside for now."

I'd already described so much of it that there wasn't a whole lot more to say other than to point out where Jesus stood in the corner and to reflect on my miracle. I never got tired of it and neither did they.

When I looked at the time, I shivered. One o'clock. The time it all started.

When I finally said good night, gave everybody their last hugs, and closed the door, I didn't have a lot of strength left, but I knew what Jesus wanted me to do. He wanted me to visit with him on my deck.

Standing in front of the rail where I'd so often sat, I looked at the stars from a whole new position, and my eyes blurred with tears.

Oh, Jesus, thank you again for my miracle.

Crisp and clear as the air itself, Jesus whispered back something I'll never forget: "Ema, thank *you* for accepting my miracle."

Christmas Day

December 25, 2011

Jason and Jeff arrived at ten on Christmas Day.

"Long time no see," I said. They wanted to arrive before Cathy so they could see the shock on her face.

Without fuss, they set up my wheelchair the same way I'd set it up the night before — right in front of my kitchen door. Then they looked at the clock.

Cathy would be all set to take me to the Salvation Army, but for once I'd have to break our tradition. I wasn't quite ready for it. Besides, I wanted to show Daddy my Christmas miracle.

Jason turned to Jeff. "She's coming! Let's walk on both sides of her in case she faints."

While they hurried out to meet her, I hid behind the Christmas tree. When was the last time I'd been this close to the star? Too long ago to remember. I pressed my teeth together when I heard them tromp up the ramp. Seconds later, Cathy's matter-of-fact chatter turned into a loud gasp. She must have seen my empty wheelchair.

"Oh, my gosh! Where's Ema?"

I pictured her crossing her arms and giving Jeff and Jason a stern look.

"It's okay," Jeff assured her.

"What do you mean, it's okay? If Ema got a new wheelchair, I'd be the first to know about it. What aren't you telling me?"

"Things have changed," Jason said.

"Well, I know that," she said. "When I called R&S to say Merry Christmas, I heard that Ema canceled. Will somebody *please* tell me what's going on? You're creeping me out."

When nobody said anything, Cathy walked from the kitchen to the archway. My heart pounded as she stepped closer. I could now see her through the branches. When she turned in my direction, I stepped out.

"Merry Christmas!"

She jumped back, stunned. Before she could fall, I grabbed her into a hug. Pulling back to see me, her jaw looked like it couldn't close. I hugged her again until my tears drenched her shoulder. A thousand nightmares, that's how many we'd been through together, and this moment made up for them all. Cathy took a full look at me. "What ... happened?"

I glanced at the boys and it started all over again: my ridiculous attempt to explain the unexplainable, to sound natural about the supernatural. Obviously Cathy believed me. How could she not when I'd never once lied to her and the miraculous proof stood eye to eye right in front of her?

She talked slowly as she shook her head. "This is crazy." She'd seen God intervene many times over the years, but this was different. This miracle totally took God outside the box. For one thing, we normally think of Jesus as practically frozen in position somewhere in heaven. We don't think of him as physically going anywhere or doing anything. We certainly don't expect him to show up in our homes—especially to someone as plain and ordinary as me: Ema McKinley from Rochester, Minnesota.

Cathy brought her hand to her forehead. "It's hard to wrap my brain around this."

I laughed. "You and me both." It excited me to think about how much this would strengthen her faith—and mine.

She pulled out her phone. "I need to take a picture to show my husband."

Quickly patting my tears, I posed beside her in front of the tree.

"Jesus . . ." I said, smiling. Somehow, it felt more appropriate to say his name than "cheese."

"There," Cathy said a few seconds later. "I texted my husband the photo. He's so going to freak out."

I clasped my hands together and looked at Jeff and Jason. "I can't wait to see Daddy."

"Okay," Jeff said. "Let's do it."

As they helped me down the ramp toward Cathy's car, I wondered what it would feel like after all these years to ride as a regular passenger. Would I even be able to sit still?

They watched me lower myself to sit shotgun beside Cathy. It felt strangely wonderful. As Cathy pulled out of the driveway, she looked extra focused.

Jason chuckled. "You don't need to grip the wheel so tight."

I suppose he had a good point. Cathy did look quite tense — almost like she was taking her driver's test or something. Then, when she put on the brakes, she threw her arm in front of me as if I might fall out.

Jason didn't let up on her. "You're driving like there's a newborn in the car."

"Enough," Cathy said. "I'm taking extra precautions because we have precious cargo up here, all right?"

My laughter flowed freely. All I knew was I never wanted to sit back there again. From now on I'd be an upright front-seat girl. Turning left and right, I devoured every last detail of scenery. Normally, I could see only the sky, boring rooftops, and treetops, but now I could see every kind of shape and living color imaginable. A whole new world. All the things I missed during my bent-over years suddenly sprang to life.

"Look at the buildings," I said, pointing out the window. "I've never seen them before. They're so beautiful. Oh, and look at those houses. Those children by that fire hydrant." On and on I went.

The very act of looking added to my feeling of transformation. Not only had God given me new body parts, he'd also given me a whole new perspective. I'd never take it for granted. It was all too good.

My heart picked up when I thought about seeing Daddy. "Do you think we'll get there before Murray comes home from church? I'd kinda like to surprise Daddy first, before my brother gets home."

"Ah, I don't think so," Jason said, "because Murray's behind us. I just saw him turn onto the road a few cars back. But don't worry. Cathy can pull into the driveway, and I'll run over and talk to Murray."

While Cathy parked, I ducked, and we all waited anxiously for Jason to come back.

"What did you tell him?" I asked as Jason opened my door.

"Just that we have a surprise for Grandpa, and could he please drive around the block for ten minutes or so."

My heart pounded as Jason helped me out of the car. I glanced toward the living room, and there sat Daddy beside his little wooden table, his back to the window. I wanted to hug him so bad it hurt.

Jeff rushed ahead to holler inside, "Hey, Grandpa, we have a surprise for you!"

I hadn't attempted stairs, and Murray had a few at his house. I wouldn't let that stop me though. I grabbed Jason and Cathy and together we struggled our way up, one step at a time. Somehow Daddy had already made it to the doorway. A smile crinkled his face as recognition flashed in his eyes.

"Daddy!"

The one who had watched me take my first toddler steps now reached out with his long farmer arms to help me up the rest of the way.

"It's okay," I said, gripping Cathy's arm. "I can do this."

I felt like pinching myself. I could now share my miracle with the man who went all those extra miles for me after Eddie left. The man who had been faithful to pray and encourage me like nobody else. Now that I had my mobility back, I practically exploded with ideas of how I could return his kindness.

Face-to-face, I threw my arms around him, crying all over again. "Merry Christmas, Daddy! Jesus healed me!"

After a good, long hug, we helped each other into the living room. It tickled me how he made sure we sat next to each other. He grabbed my hand and wouldn't let go, not for a second. Wow, I loved this incredible man. The way he held on tight reminded me how he'd always been there, protecting and caring for me all those years.

After a bit of talking and sharing, we heard a voice. "Is it safe to come in yet?" Murray. I'd almost forgotten about him. Whoops. We took over his house, and here he waited patiently and unruffled.

Jason helped me to my feet so I could walk, bend, and show Murray my hands and feet. "Look what Jesus did!"

His eyes bugged out and I burst out laughing.

"Have a seat," I said. "Boy, do I have a story to tell you."

Surprise!

I hid behind the curtain in Dr. Bell's office, listening to Jason and Cathy whisper on the bench by the window.

Come on, Dr. Bell. After all the ups and downs we'd been through together, I couldn't wait to show him the new me. A light knock on the door sent my heart racing, and I heard him step in. Slowly and carefully, I peered through the curtain as he took a seat by his computer.

"How are you guys doing?"

"All right," Jason said as casually as ever.

"So you're here for a question-and-answer appointment about Ema. How's she doing?"

"Great," Cathy said. "Surprisingly well, actually."

The room stayed quiet as Dr. Bell pulled up something on the screen.

How would he handle seeing me? Would he look like the nurses whose jaws dropped open? Hopefully, the nurses had respected my wishes and kept quiet about this. I wanted Dr. Bell to be completely and a hundred percent shocked out of his mind.

Unable to wait a second longer, I tore back the curtain and took a few steps forward.

Dr. Bell froze in disbelief. "Please tell me Ema has a twin."

"Nope." I laughed. "It's me. Ever since my Christmas miracle."

He brought a hand to his forehead. "Christmas miracle?"

"Don't worry, I'll tell you everything." And I did too, starting from the beginning with my wheelchair falling over. Dr. Bell's eyes stayed glued on me, stunned but thirsty for every last word.

When Cathy signaled to Jason to pull out his phone, I said, "Mind if we take a picture?"

Dr. Bell threw up his arms. "Why not?"

I wobbled over confidently and wrapped my arm around him while Jason clicked.

"Well, what do you think?" I said.

Dr. Bell laughed. "What do I think? I think this has nothing to do with medical science. It's a total act of God."

Later, Dr. Bell, my primary-care doctor, wrote an official statement:

Nearly 20 years ago, Ema was diagnosed with Complex Regional Pain Syndrome, an uncommon disorder of amplified musculoskeletal pain and disability that can develop after an injury. Since that time she has suffered complications of severe widespread pain, disability, and skin problems, for which she has undergone treatment. For years she was confined to a wheelchair, unable to stand or walk.

Early on Christmas [Eve] Morning, 2011, a number of her symptoms improved dramatically—most notably her ability to straighten herself, rise up from her wheelchair, and walk a short distance. While she still experiences a number of symptoms, her overall condition is significantly better.

Sudden, unforeseen improvements after years of pain and disability have been reported only rarely in cases such as Ema's. While I currently cannot offer a clear medical explanation for her dramatic improvement, and cannot speculate regarding other possible interpretations, I am nonetheless delighted with Ema's recent progress. Along with all of her care team, I share in her hope for continued improvement.

DAVID BELL, M.D., MAYO CLINIC

January 31, 2012

Cathy, Jason, and I stopped in front of Dr. Bengston's office and peered through the glass beside his open door. I nodded at Jason and he started his video recording.

Dr. Bengston looked at the papers in his hand, unaware he was being watched. When he moved closer, I thought for sure he'd see me, but he didn't. Instead, he dropped a few sheets in the recycle bin and studied the remaining ones in his hands.

Okay, so that didn't work. On to plan B. I planted myself in his doorway. He looked over and did a double take. About time. He walked over to me with eyes as big as his laughter.

And I laughed with him. Especially when he shook his head and set his hand on my shoulder.

"I can't believe you're standing here." He wrapped me in a good-natured hug and stepped back so he could look me up and down. "It's good to see you. I've heard about you. You look fantastic!"

"What? You heard about it?" My heart sank. Who in the world had told him? Nobody was supposed to breathe a word.

"How do you feel?" he asked.

"Like a brand-new person."

Smiling, he pulled off his glasses and stuck one of the ends in his mouth. "Get out of here," he mumbled. His eyes twinkled above his widening smile, but he looked mystified. I'd never seen him like this. Speechless.

I snickered. "I'm literally like a brand-new person."

He pulled his glasses out of his mouth and dragged the other end across his chin. "Oh, my gosh, you look great!"

I beamed. "And this has only been since Christmas Eve day!"

He shook his head. "Your coloring and everything has changed. Do you know that? I mean, everything! Wow!"

"So here we have a straight foot and we have a straight hand with new skin on it too." He moved closer and touched my hand as I continued. "We also have a spine that is no longer this way."

He crossed his arms and uncrossed them, astounded. I stood my straightest, relishing the facts as I opened them like gift-wrapped presents. "This all happened on Christmas Eve morning."

He snapped his fingers. "So it happened — boom — just like that?"

I shrugged. "Well, when God shows up, things happen."

"Amazing. Like a bolt of lightning. And you'd fallen?"

I leaned in, frustrated. "Did someone tip you off?"

He turned his back to me for a second before shifting to face me again. "I'm trying to think who talked to me about this. I can't remember who . . ."

Miffed, I turned to Jason, who was still recording. "Shoot, someone told!"

Dr. Bengston laughed but didn't say anything.

"You should have seen when all the nurses came out," I said. "They nearly passed out when they saw me. And all the therapists." I giggled with delight.

He leaned on the doorframe, staring and beaming. "How do you feel?"

"Amazing. I'm still having pain, but it's nothing like before."

He nodded. "Where does it hurt?"

"Mostly in my back and lower hips."

"Okay," he said. "Well, let's take a look . . ."

February 14, 2012

My next victim was Dr. Arora. I'd worked it out with his nurse in advance, but when I arrived at the nurses' station, it took a good five minutes before everybody calmed down enough so we could get to business. Meantime, Cathy pointed her camera at each of their surprised faces.

One of Dr. Arora's nurses said, "Ready? We can go in now." She led me to a room I'd never been in. I hid behind the door. Nobody made a peep because we could hear Dr. Arora on the other side of it. The more I tried to listen, the more I caught his ruffled tone. I'd never heard him like this before. So intense.

"What do you mean Ema's in there? She couldn't be. She doesn't fit."

I cupped a hand over my mouth. This was Dr. Arora, my all-time favorite bright bow-tie doctor — and he was arguing about whether or not I could fit through the door. I felt like I was about to explode with excitement. After years of benefiting from his fun-loving personality and encouragement, I'd finally be able to give him something valuable in return: the gift of my miracle.

He knocked quick and opened the door. I held my breath, knowing he'd face my empty wheelchair in the middle of the room. The door closed, and at last he saw me standing there, grinning from ear to ear. Jason started capturing the moment on his phone.

Without batting an eyelash, Dr. Arora threw his hand over his mouth. I couldn't help myself — I burst out laughing. I'd never seen his eyes so wide, his mouth so open. He looked from my face to my feet, then back to my face.

"Wha-what happened? What did you do?" Angling his head, he pulled me into a hug, then backed away and crossed his arms, staring and shaking his head from side to side. "Ema, I'm so happy!"

I chuckled. "You know that crooked spine ... and the hand that wouldn't open?"

"Yeah, yeah, yeah, I know!"

"And the crooked foot and everything?" I continued.

He quickly scratched his head. "Yeah, yeah, yeah, I know!"

I pointed to each of my body parts. "I have a new foot. I have a new hand. And my spine is straight. My neck is straight."

He stepped closer and got real quiet. "What did you do?"

"I didn't do anything. What doctors couldn't do in almost nineteen years, Jesus showed up and did in just a few minutes."

He looked from me to the empty wheelchair and flopped against the wall. His voice stayed quiet. "What happened?"

I held out my hand so he could take a good look. "Jesus literally opened up my hand and straightened it out. I just stared at the palm of my hand. At the open, raw creases. At the blood red lines. Then, within seconds, I saw new flesh growing over all the raw parts of my hand."

"This is fabulous," he whispered slowly. "This is so ..."

"Jesus started on my neck, then on my spine, and the next thing I knew, I was lying flat on the floor with a straight back!"

"Well, you look wonderful," he said. "But when?"

Cathy spoke up. "Christmas Eve morning. It all started when she accidentally fell out of her chair and ended up lying on the floor for several hours."

His eyebrows shot up and he gave me one of the most endearing smiles I'd ever seen. One I'll truly never forget.

March 30, 2012

When I called Dr. Otley's nurse, Becky, and told her I could walk now because God healed me, surprise filled her voice.

"Um, Dr. Otley probably needs to see you as soon as possible," she said. "Could you come in this Friday? We'll make sure we get you in between appointments."

Jason wouldn't be able to come because Connor was scheduled for surgery, but Cathy could take me, so ... "Friday's fine," I told her.

When I arrived, Dr. Otley's nurses clamored around in shock and amazement. I doubted I'd ever get used to this. Several took turns hugging me. "I know you told me about this on the phone," Becky said, "but seeing you standing here ... well, it's amazing."

I followed her to a procedure room, a larger room where light fixtures hung over the bed and instruments lay covered beneath a long piece of cloth. I'd always disliked this kind of room because it reminded me how they wanted to amputate my leg. Right now, however, it reminded me how God wanted to spare it. And it reminded me of something else too. My right leg was the first one to touch the floor when Jesus floated me to my feet. A small detail, but like everything else, it amazed me no end.

I slid behind the curtain that divided the room and lowered myself onto the bench to wait.

"Ready for me to get him?" Becky asked. "I want to be here too so I can see the look on his face."

"Go for it," I said. And with that, she pulled back the curtain to hide me. My mind tripped back to the doctor who said, "You mean you wouldn't amputate your leg to save your life?" My scars were silent reminders of that trial. And I'd always like my heart-shaped scar the most.

The door creaked open. "Hello? Is Ema in here?"

Dr. Otley didn't waste time before his hand curled around my curtain. Pulling it back, the world stopped. His jaw dropped and his saucer-wide eyes became glassy. He looked almost dizzy with shock. It's a good thing I'd stayed in a sitting position because if *this* freaked him out, what would have happened if I'd been standing from the get-go? Cathy snapped a picture, capturing both Dr. Otley and Becky.

"Look," I said, wiggling my feet. "No more hanging off my wheelchair."

He started to sob. Now this ... I had not expected. Cathy and I looked at each other, not knowing what to do, so we cried right along with him. She grabbed my hands and helped me to my feet. This just about did him in.

"Are you for real?" he said, closely eyeing me. "I've just got to feel you." He grabbed my shoulders, patted my head and face, and pinched my cheeks.

Laughter spilled out of me. "I had a miracle."

"I can see that. I mean, what else could it be? And your legs? I've got to look at them and feel them."

Cathy and I had never seen him like this. What did he think— that I had a fake foot sticking out of my pants or something? I stuck out my leg. "Check it out. I've got a brand-new straight foot. Jesus showed up and did this. He did all of it."

He grabbed my hand, my foot, and my cheeks. "Astounding . . ."

"I want to know about this. All of it." He turned to Becky. "Please cancel my next appointment. Ema and I need to talk." He reached for my hand. "Now tell me about this from the beginning. I want to know all about your miracle and what Jesus is like."

Outreach

My miracle launched me into a whole new type of busy. To work on my balance, I saw Dr. Kathryn Stolp, a wonderful doctor in physical therapy. Thankfully, she started me off slowly, but best of all, she listened to me. She knew how much I wanted to step out into the community and show everybody the new me.

Wherever I went, people did double takes. So many remembered me as the crooked lady, the smiling woman who hung awkwardly off her wheelchair all those years. Naturally, people wanted to stop and ask questions, even at the Rochester Athletic Club where I regularly walked the track.

A middle-aged lady caught up with me. "Do I know you?"

"It's possible," I said. "You might have seen me when I was crooked and bent over in my wheelchair."

"Oh, my gosh! That's it. What happened to you?"

"Well, let me tell you ..."

I burst with joy as I filled in the dots about this God story. I'd always been close to Jesus, but my miracle made each emotion and interaction that much more over the top.

As I sat down in the athletic club's reception area with Jason and Cathy, something else struck me. I stared wide-eyed at the two of them as tears filled my eyes.

My wheelchair. I don't know why I hadn't thought about this before. When I'd walked out of my office with Jesus, I'd left my tipped-over wheelchair on the floor, right where I fell out of it. After

Jesus left my bedroom, I'd gone to different rooms trying out the new me, but I didn't touch anything in my office. And later, I shifted all my attention to the boys because I wanted a creative idea to surprise them with my miracle. Nothing came to me until they arrived. That's when I hurried to my office as fast as my wobbly legs could carry me and quickly grabbed the handles of my wheelchair to push it down the hall.

"What is it?" Jason said, staring back at me. "You look like you're somewhere else."

"My wheelchair," I said, shaking my head. "I just thought of something. After my miracle, I never picked it up off the floor. Jesus did."

The gravity of my words sunk into their faces. I was weak and off balance that day. Picking up the wheelchair would have been extremely difficult for me. I would have at least remembered it.

"It had to be Jesus," I said. "That's how I was able to grab it so fast when I pushed it to the kitchen."

They entered the aftershock of this unforgettable detail. In the midst of Jesus giving me this most amazing miracle, he had even cared enough to pick up the pieces.

Armed with this new realization, when family members came over, I joked about how Jesus helped me clean my office. "He picked up my chair," I told my cousins.

If my aunts, uncles, and cousins tired of hearing me go on, they never showed it. In fact, some, like Jim, my cousin Linda Bauer's husband, couldn't get enough of my story. After he'd pondered and probed it one day, he grabbed my Bible off the end table and started flipping through like he was on a treasure hunt. "Ema, I'd like to read you a passage from Luke 13:10–13."

"Go for it," I said.

"On a Sabbath Jesus was teaching in one of the synagogues, and a woman was there who had been crippled by a spirit for eighteen years. She was bent over and could not straighten up at all. When Jesus saw her, he called her forward and said to her, 'Woman, you are set free from your infirmity.' Then he put his hands on her, and immediately she straightened up and praised God."

Jim set the Bible aside and gazed at me in the solemn space of the moment. He didn't need to say anything because the text spoke for itself. Two thousand years after it was written, Jesus had performed a miracle similar to the one he'd done with the crooked lady in the Bible—only this time, he'd done it with me! And Jesus had given us both our miracles on a Saturday. What an amazing, changeless God to reach out across the generations and heal his daughters.

My future may be uncertain, but more than ever, I knew Jesus would help me face my fears.

October 17, 2012

As much as I dreaded it, I wanted to go off that horrible morphine. Jason and Cathy sat across from me in my living room when I opened the topic.

"But you're still having a lot of pain," Jason said. "And what about the drug withdrawals?"

Bingo. He'd hit on the area that scared me most. We all knew how horrible and deadly those withdrawals could be.

"God will give me the courage," I said. "He'll help me through."

Cathy looked unsure. "What do you want us to do?"

"Well, for one thing, I want someone to be with me 24-7. I don't want to take any chances."

I knew I couldn't go off it all at once. A few months earlier, under the direction of Dr. Bell, I'd reduced my morphine from 2000 to 1600 milligrams, so I thought it made sense to reduce it by 300 milligrams a week. That was aggressive by normal standards, which is probably why, a couple weeks later, I had my first hallucination.

I'd never had a hallucination all those years on the morphine. Now, as I went off it so quickly, I got hit in the middle of the night.

"Stop!" hollered Cathy, grabbing my arms. "Where are you going?"

"Outside!" I shouted, trying to fling my leg onto my bedroom windowsill.

"Not that way, you don't. Let's get you back into bed."

"But the house is on fire!" I shouted.

A few hours later, when Cathy told me what happened, I couldn't believe it. "Praise God for his protection," I said. Thankfully, it happened only once. Just enough to give me a small taste of what God had protected me from all those years.

From that day on, I reduced my morphine by only 100 milligrams a week. I still had to go through that whole sweating and shaking thing, but at least I could see the light at the end of the tunnel.

February 2013

When I answered the phone, a woman introduced herself as Melinda. "I'm from the Madonna Towers nursing home. Your hairdresser told me about your amazing story, and I was wondering if you'd mind sharing it with our residents."

A fountain of excitement welled up in me. Of course I'd do it. Why not? It would give me another opportunity to encourage people.

While I prepared the points for my talk, the miracle struck me all over again. Would I ever stop feeling overwhelmed by it?

Straightening my red blazer, I walked onto the platform with Cathy at my side. I wasn't nervous. My shakes were just the tail end of the morphine withdrawal. I'd always enjoyed public speaking, even back in high school. And what a joy to stand in front of a group on my own two feet!

I looked into the eyes of each precious person, and there was

Bill Butts, my R&S driver. He must have heard about it from Cathy. *Thank you, Jesus, for the surprise.*

From the moment I opened my mouth, my story flowed out, from accident to miracle. My heart soared, and I could tell from people's faces that they were soaring right along with me. My talk felt like a wild ride. Like I sat at the front of a roller coaster, leading the way through all the ups and downs. Toward the end of our time together, I shared some advice:

"You don't ever want to give up. Oh, my goodness, people. Jesus is so real. Make him a part of your day. Talk to him. Build a relationship with him. I don't know anybody who could stand up to that level of pain and suffering without him. You just can't. That kind of strength comes only from Jesus. It comes from asking him and trusting him every single day. Sometimes our hearts are literally broken with pain. But let me tell you, precious people, there's only one person who can mend a shattered heart, and that's Jesus. Call on him as your lifetime friend. He'll never leave you."

I searched their faces. Several sat in wheelchairs. One wore a mask over his mouth. Another had tubes in her nose. Each person reminded me of where I'd come from before Jesus healed me. An older gentleman in a gray suit looked attentive but lonely.

"Everyone in this room has problems," I said, "but Jesus is the solution. Don't let anybody cheat you out of having the best day possible. We all have hurts. We all have trying times. Before we started, Melinda shared with me that her mom has cancer. That's not too big for Jesus — but we do need to stay close to him. He's worth every bit of our praise and love, dear friends. And he's waiting to give you peace and joy for your journey. The rewards in the end are going to be so awesome."

I smiled at a young nurse who was beside a man in a wheelchair. "Be bold for Jesus. Put yourself out there and tell everybody how much you love Jesus and what he means to you. I still have RSD. I still have it in my feet as I'm standing here. I still have it in my hands.

I even have it in my teeth, and it feels like an abscessed tooth. The pain never goes away, but I tell you what ... I don't sweat the small stuff anymore—not when I'm on my feet and walking forward."

I looked at Melinda. "Thank you for asking me to share today. And I pray each one of you finds yourself a little closer to Jesus. When things get tough, take hold of his hand and let him show you how much he loves you. He waits to be your helper each moment of the day. Thank you."

The room erupted into applause, and Cathy stepped up to the platform to help me down. I could hardly wait to greet everybody.

That older gentleman in the gray suit squeezed my hand extra tight. "I'd give anything if my wife could have heard you today."

"Why couldn't she?" I asked.

He looked at the floor. "Because the flu's going around on her wing, and they had to quarantine everybody."

Instantly, I felt that all-too-familiar tug of the Holy Spirit, and I knew what he wanted me to do and say. "Flu or no flu, I'd love to visit your wife."

"You'd do that?" He studied me. "Well, that would be wonderful!"

Before we could talk ourselves out of it, Jason, Cathy, and I followed the man to the elevator and all the way up to his wife's little room.

"Mabel, we have visitors. I brought that same lady who spoke downstairs. She wanted to see you."

Mabel sat tall and straight in her wheelchair. With the tracheotomy tube in place, she couldn't speak, but her eyes flickered bright as candles when she saw me.

I grabbed her hand. "So honored to meet you." She nodded and I went right to my story about what Jesus did for me. Tears streamed down her face, and I was powerless to do anything except inwardly give thanks.

This is what it's all about, isn't it, Father? You tell us what to do and you give us the strength to do it. Please give me more opportunities to make a difference.

Recovery

June 2013

I nearly dropped the phone when a woman from the Salvation Army asked if I'd go to the Twin Cities and speak to a big group of men in an addiction recovery program. God had given me more opportunities than expected. I'd already shared my miracle in nursing homes, women's groups, youth groups, on the radio, and even on international TV— but could I really share it with men in recovery? It seemed like a stretch.

"Thanks for asking," I said. "I'll get back to you." After I hung up, I offered a quick prayer and called Dr. Cindy.

"What do I know about talking to addicts?" I said. "I've never walked that road."

"Let's think about this," Dr. Cindy said. "I believe I know somebody who's been through some pretty horrible circumstances and drug withdrawals."

Her words sank in ... and turned on a light. She was absolutely right. How had I missed it? This invitation to speak to hurting men had my name written all over it—in God's handwriting.

While I paced the floor praying, God told me he wanted me to do something a little different. He wanted me to take my talk to the next level and introduce these men to my best friend—to the One who kept me alive so I could be standing in front of them.

231

I thanked God that I felt so much better since coming off the morphine. I'd also just received a good report. Apart from the old stomach issues, the rest of my body didn't show any morphine damage. To the doctor's delight, even my liver looked great. Hearing such good news made me all the more eager to tell these men my story.

I looked at the clock. Ten minutes until starting—but where were all the people? Sadly, most of the one hundred and fifty chairs were still empty.

That's okay, I told myself. The day is in God's hands.

Father, thank you for each hurting person you send my way. May everything go just the way you want it—even if I end up just talking to a few.

I looked at the floor as I continued to pace and pray. I wanted God to open their minds to hear his truth. He loved these people, and I wanted him to love them through me. After several minutes, I looked up—and lo and behold, the chairs were mostly filled. I couldn't have been happier.

The men represented several nationalities and age groups, but my eyes kept returning to a man in his early twenties. Gina, who had asked me to speak, stepped up and introduced me.

I looked at the crowd. "Thank you. It's great to be here today. I'd like to start off by asking for a volunteer." I turned to Gina. "Would you mind helping me pick one?"

"How about Nate," she said, pointing to the same young man I'd been noticing. This told me God was up to something.

"Come on up, Nate. Thanks for helping. I'd like you to try something that's really quite difficult, but I know you can do it." I nodded toward my wheelchair, which we'd brought to the front as a prop. "I'd like you to sit in my wheelchair and position yourself in something close to a ninety-degree angle."

He scrunched his face with uncertainty. Then he struggled his way over. He didn't quite get there, but at least he looked noticeably uncomfortable.

"Good. Now I'd like you to tuck your left foot under the footrest."
He raised an eyebrow but did it anyway.

"Nate, I'd like you to stay there for a bit while I talk to your friends."

"Okay," he said weakly.

And I turned my attention back to the men so I could tell them about my accident. As expected, Nate lasted only about five minutes before he looked extremely uncomfortable.

"Go ahead and sit up," I said, ignoring a couple laughs and snickers. "How do you feel?"

Relief washed over him as he stretched left and right. "My neck's hurting pretty bad. My back's totally stiff, and my knee's kinda cramped."

"I believe it," I said. "And that's only after five minutes. Can you imagine what it would have felt like to sit like that for fifteen years, 24-7?"

His eyes widened. "No, ma'am. I can't."

I thanked him, and he more than happily returned to his seat.

As I bled out my story, I watched the men's faces. I could almost see the Lord speaking to their hearts. I loved every minute, loved seeing the Lord redeem my pain.

A hush fell over the room when Jason flashed pictures on the screen of my deformed hand and foot as well as my crooked neck and spine. When I told them how the doctor had me on 2000 milligrams of morphine, their jaws dropped.

"I know what it's like to go through two horrific drug withdrawals," I said. "One nearly took my life — but God wasn't finished with me yet. I also know what it's like to be hit with severe depression. I felt like I went to hell and back, but I didn't need to stay there. From my pit, God reminded me that I could turn around. And he helped me tell myself, *Be thankful in spite of how you feel. You're better and stronger than this.*

"Friends, that's what I want to tell you. God's love is stronger than any fear. Stronger than any addiction or hold the enemy has on your life. I called out to Jesus, and you can do the same. God wants to help each one of you."

What was going on? I saw tears in their eyes. These were big, tough men. A few of them turned to the guys beside them and gave them a big side hug. We all felt it, this powerful connection. This God-sized moment where our broken pieces somehow intersected.

"This isn't just my miracle," I told them. "It's your miracle too. And it's a miracle you can share with others because we all need this kind of hope and encouragement. This life is full of mind-blowing hurts and suffering, but you can give it to Jesus, and he'll give you all the strength you need. And when you give your old twisted life to God, let me tell you, friends, it's absolutely gone. Your past is wiped clean, and God completely straightens you out—just like he straightened me out.

"Jesus, the same God-man who gave up his life for you two thousand years ago, wants to give you a brand-new heart tonight. And a brand-new life. When you say 'yes' to Jesus, you can ask him for guidance, and he'll direct you. You can ask him for strength, and he'll help you make the right decisions. Even if you fail—because we all do—he'll be right there waiting for you to take hold of his hand. And he'll be waiting to pick you up and help you walk forward."

I gripped the podium as I searched their faces.

Lord, this is your moment. Please move by the power of your Holy Spirit.

"Is there anyone here who would like to know this same Jesus who showed up in my room and straightened my foot, opened my palm, and literally got down on one knee and asked for my hand? Maybe you made a commitment to him in the past, but you haven't been following him or making the right decisions. If you'd like to follow him today or renew your commitment, I invite you to come down to the front and do it now."

In less than thirty seconds, forty-five or fifty guys surrounded me at the front. And miracle of miracles, God held me together as I prayed for the whole big group of them: *"Jesus, I'm ready to commit my life to you and receive a brand-new heart. Thank you for forgiving my sins. I'm ready to partner with you and have a brand-new start. In Jesus' name. Amen."*

Other than the night when I saw Jesus himself, I'd never seen anything so moving. Then came the hugs and thank-yous before Gina hurried over. "When can we have you back?"

She said a few other things, but I got distracted when I noticed three new guys walk in. To my delight, four of the men who had just heard my talk rushed over to the newcomers. When one leaned over like he was me in a wheelchair, I knew he was describing my story. These men hadn't even left the building, and here they were, taking me up on my challenge to share God's awesome miracle.

I waved when one of them pointed in my direction. After so many years of being pointed at and singled out, I couldn't think of a better kind of finger-pointing. Well, I can tell you one thing: As long as I have breath, I'll keep pointing my finger right back to my Maker.

To God be the glory!

And why wouldn't I keep pointing to him? My whole tragic story and life-changing miracle had been all about him from the beginning. My Jesus, my Savior, my lifeline—my rock. Whether I could see him with my eyes or feel him like a rush of heaven was beside the point. Because Immanuel, God with us, would always live up to his name and be with me forever.

> *He lifted me out of the slimy pit, out of the mud and mire; he set my feet on a rock and gave me a firm place to stand.*
>
> PSALM 40:2

Ema's Heart

Three times I pleaded with the Lord to take it away
from me. But he said to me, "My grace is sufficient
for you, for my power is made perfect in weakness."

2 CORINTHIANS 12:8−9

Dear Friends,

Like many of you, I still deal with pain and weakness, and I need to draw on God's strength every day.

Perhaps he will heal me completely and the RSD will go away for good. Then again, maybe he'll wait until heaven. But no matter what happens, our good and loving God has good and loving reasons for everything he allows into our lives.

I can't thank him enough for showing up and giving me my mobility back. I'm still overwhelmed by my miracle, and it sure helps me keep going.

Some days are flat out hard. Daddy died this past year. So did Max and Savannah. Sometimes I feel that lonesome nagging ache. That's when I turn to God in the secret place. I reach out for him with all my heart and see him quietly, actively at work.

I pray you do too.

If you've asked God for healing and nothing has happened, please don't be discouraged. I prayed for healing for eighteen and a half years before God gave me my miracle—and I still keep praying for healing.

We must never doubt God's incredibly big love for us. It

helps us rejoice when we remember he has the big picture in mind, and he never wastes our pain.

Sometimes I think God allows suffering to help us focus on our eternal home. Our circumstances are temporary compared to the glory that will soon be revealed in us. This life is actually just a stepping-stone. In heaven, when we see Jesus face-to-face, we'll be a hundred percent healed and whole.

I don't know what you're going through, but I do know that God hasn't forgotten you. It may *feel* like it, but Jesus is just as much for you as he is for me. He loves each one of us equally, and he'll be faithful to carry you too.

I pray this book has been an oasis in your desert — because you mean everything to him. Thank you so very much for letting me share my heart.

Love,

Ema

Praise be to the God and Father of our Lord Jesus Christ, the Father of compassion and the God of all comfort, who comforts us in all our troubles, so that we can comfort those in any trouble with the comfort we ourselves receive from God.

2 CORINTHIANS 1:3–4

Epilogue

Ema McKinley

"I know the perfect person to write your story."

When anchorwoman Betsy Singer explained her words, I added Cheryl Ricker to my growing list of possible writers. Several other authors had approached me about writing a book, so more than ever, I needed divine direction on which one to pick.

God, I think you're going to have to hit me on the side of the head about this one.

When Cheryl left a message on my answering machine, I fell in love with her sweet, young voice. A little later, as we sat across from each other at the Rochester Athletic Club Café, I wasn't afraid to tell her so.

We had a great time getting to know each other. I'd already checked out her blog, and I loved that she wrote poetry ... like me. She'd written a Zondervan gift book, *A Friend in the Storm*, which showed we had the same heart—to share God's hope and encouragement. Still, this huge decision had to be more than an emotional or logical one. It had to be a Jesus one.

When Cheryl told me that her agent, Alice Crider, wanted to fly in to Rochester to meet me, I agreed to spend several hours with the two of them at Cheryl's home. I loved every moment, but I didn't hear from God—until five days later.

While out on my deck praying at three o'clock in the morning, I had another Jesus moment. And the Lord spoke to me as clear as the stars: *"Pick Cheryl Ricker."*

It hit me so fast that I whipped around and fell on the hard deck floor. In pain but too excited to care, I crawled back inside, laughing and crying at the same time. I finally had my answer!

In order to surprise Cheryl with the news, I needed Betsy Singer's help. I asked her to call Cheryl and plan for the two of them to get together at the café.

Twenty minutes into their visit, I walked in with a dozen red roses. "Congratulations! God picked you to write the book." I wrapped my shocked new friend in a long, tight hug, and God's been hugging us together ever since.

Jesus flung open the door for this book because he believes in it and because it isn't just my miracle. It's yours too. God bless you!

CHERYL RICKER

Thank you to all my prayer warriors who lifted me up as I wrote.

Alice, thanks for believing in me from day one.

John, Jane, and Bob, it has been a joy to work with you on this project. God truly answered my prayer when I asked him to provide the best possible editors.

Dwight, what a husband you are. I can't thank you enough for standing by my side day and night. After transcribing endless hours of interviews, you became my tireless cheerleader, helping me every step of the way.

Jesus, thank you. Thank you for whispering my name in Ema's keen ear. My life is forever changed by this beautiful woman of God and her awe-inspiring story.

Thank you for connecting the bits and pieces of this book together. May it grow wings and fly into your mission field, wherever you want it to go for your glory.

May love be the loudest voice in this story so minds and hearts open freely to your life-changing presence and grace.

In Tune

When you call Me, I will answer;
I will calm you to the quick.
I feel deep inside each flattening ache
that leaves your insides sick.

Since I made you in My power,
not one cell, synapse or nerve,
not one groaning of your spirit
ever passes Me unheard.

CHERYL RICKER, *A Friend in the Storm*

My Medical
and Legal Records

You may embrace my story with childlike faith because you know God can do anything—*or* you may question and clamor for evidence, like a lawyer reaching for facts. That's fine. Like any good lawyer, you don't want to trust the testimony of just one witness, especially when that witness is a sixty-seven-year-old woman who's taken a lot of pain medication. I don't blame you.

That's why God, in his wisdom, gave us many credible witnesses to this incredible miracle.

I've included written comments from several medical doctors, courtroom judges, my psychologist, and my attorney. These are taken directly from my medical reports and court documents. I introduce each of them with a brief summary, then I present you with official excerpts from my documented records.

I share these reports with deep gratitude for my doctors and therapists, who persevered through my incurable condition with the best possible care available at that time. May their expert "testimony" below shine more light on your path.

Author's Note: Nothing has been added except bold letters for emphasis ☺.

On January 26, 1995, I signed a retainer agreement with my lawyer, Charlie Bird, for my Workers' Compensation claim. He went right to work on my case, collecting information and sending me for medical exams. A report from Dr. Noll on October 24, 1995, details a physical-therapy exam that shows the extent of my disability.

> Mrs. McKinley had a recurrence of her symptoms and find-ings, beginning in September 1994 ... Because she had failed invasive measures during her first course of reflex sympathetic dystrophy, we were hesitant to employ these measures with her recurrence. She did, however, have a trial of modalities in phys-ical therapy, medications for pain control, casting and splint-ing of the lower extremity, all of which were without benefit. Finally she had treatment in the Pain Management C[linic] (PMC), which did not alleviate her symptoms or improve her function. In fact, she complains that, following the treatment in the PMC, she has had increased pain in her shoulders, upper back, and neck with no improvement in the left leg pain.
>
> With this history and lack of response to interventions which we have recommended, I have explained to Mrs. McKinley that **I know of no other medical treatments to employ at this time and would consider her at maximal medical improve-ment ...***
>
> On examination ... **the left leg ... is held in an internally rotated and adducted position at the hip**. Passive range of motion of the left hip and knee is normal. Examination of the distal left lower extremity reveals the following: Swelling which begins below the knee, a purplish discoloration about the ankle and heel area, a cooler skin temperature to palpation about the foot, a shiny appearance to the skin over the pretibial area and dorsum of the foot, and an equino varus contracture at the ankle. **The ankle is essentially in a fixed position** and in approximately 35% of plantar flexion along with 50° of

---

* Bold added for emphasis.

foot inversion ... The tibial calcaneal angle is in approximately 40° of varus. **She is unable to bear weight on the left lower extremity and ambulates with two axillary crutches ...**

Mrs. McKinley's reflex sympathetic dystrophy was considered severe in that she is unable to weight bear to effectively perform most of the activities of daily living ...

Although my lawyer had been discussing a possible settlement with the opposing side, when he and I met on February 14, 1996, he saw my condition and realized how much I'd changed. In a letter to the opposing lawyer, he wrote:

I met with Ms. McKinley today. I am very surprised at her worsening condition. She is now in a wheelchair and there is great concern that the RSD is now progressing through the shoulder and into the neck area ...

I cannot make an offer based upon the condition set out in your letter of February 12, 1996. Dr. Bengston is quite clear that the RSD, in its entirety, is related to the work injury ... Unfortunately, this condition appears to be progressing, and **I am quite certain, at this point, that Ms. McKinley is permanently and totally disabled ...**

It is hard to describe the worsening of her condition over the months, and I think it would be beneficial for you to meet with her once again ... I think that, only in this way, can you obtain a picture of her current lifestyle and disability ...

On January 6, 1997, we received our first judgment on our workers' comp case. The judge submitted a detailed ruling that included forty-one "findings of fact." The facts were confirmed through testimony, independent medical evaluations, and my medical records. They included details about my injury, follow-up treatment, attempts to return to work, and my worsening symptoms that landed me in a wheelchair. Here are a couple of their findings:

> 23. **The parties have stipulated that the employee is permanently totally disabled**, although they disagree as to whether her work injury is a substantial cause of that disability.

> 28. The employee is permanently totally disabled as a result of her work injury of April 10, 1993.

The court ruled in my favor and ordered my employer's insurance to pay disability benefits, impairment compensation, legal fees, and other expenses. As expected, the opposing side filed an appeal. The Workers' Compensation Court of Appeals made its ruling on July 16, 1997. The key findings in the January 1997 ruling were affirmed: I had RSD, clearly caused by my work injury.

The appeals judge also addressed allegations raised by the opposing attorney that I had psychological/emotional problems before my work injury and that my RSD symptoms were caused by psychological conditions rather than my work-related injury. The appeals judge noted that "there is a lack of evidence of any of these [psychological] conditions from other medical witnesses," and then went on to state:

> After her work injury, a psychological evaluation [was] done of the employee on August 9, 1993. The assessment of this evaluation stated, '[p]sychological evaluation results in a similar impression to the psychiatric evaluation. This patient's primary source of distress at the present appears to be her pain and there is little evidence of psychological or psychiatric disorder in addition to her pain syndrome.' **The compensation judge reasonably rejected the argument that the employee's permanent total disability was substantially caused by the employee's psychological/psychiatric problems.**

Substantial evidence supports the finding that the employee is permanently and totally disabled as a result of her work injury of April 10, 1993.

In January 1998, a court settlement finally was reached. In 1999, as my condition worsened, Charlie Bird contacted my doctors, asking for medical opinions about my medical prognosis and future medical costs. On June 24, 1999, Dr. Bengston provided this opinion:

I concur that Ms. McKinley's current state of disability will likely remain unchanged for her lifetime.

On January 26, 2001, we received another settlement. Over the next couple of years, however, I continued to develop new physical problems that were due to the work-related injury and resulting RSD. The opposing side claimed the problems were not related to the injury. After reviewing about a dozen different issues, the court concluded that most of my problems were related to the RSD — medications used to treat the RSD, being wheelchair-bound, and my posture resulting from RSD. On February 3, 2004, the court made the following ruling:

It is furthered ordered that the self-insured employer shall pay for medical care related to the following conditions, as determined above: heart, skin, bladder, throat, dental, massage therapy to the right shoulder girdle, sleep problems ...

The court ruling didn't stop the continuing insurance questions regarding my medical expenses. As my RSD sores oozed and insurance balked at paying for gauze, my dermatologist, Dr. Otley, provided a letter on October 21, 2004, confirming the quantity of supplies that were needed.

Ms. Ema McKinley has reflex sympathetic dystrophy and a blistering skin eruption due to the underlying reflex sympathetic dystrophy. She requires dressing materials to care for the wounds and to absorb fluid that constantly pours out of the wounds.

The recommended wound care materials would include a tub of white petroleum jelly, which she would use one tub per week. She uses plastic Transpore tape, four rolls per day, 28 rolls per week, and 8 x 10 sterile ABD pads to absorb the extensive fluid, 60 of those per day, 420 per week. They also need sterile gloves, ten per day, or 70 per week.

Just one month later, on November 23, 2004, I had a follow-up visit with Dr. Bengston. Amazingly, the leg that the doctors wanted to amputate two months earlier had mostly healed. In his clinical note that day, Dr. Bengston wrote:

Ms. McKinley returns for her regular four-week follow-up. She has been doing well in regards to her lower extremities and that they have had almost complete resolution of the edema. There are still some scabbing lesions on the examination, but they are no longer draining any clear fluid.

The RSD sores and court battles quieted just in time for me to deal with my increasing chronic pain. Fourteen years after the accident, my medications still weren't helping much. The doctors were running out of treatment options, but thankfully, they weren't my only hope. I was dependent on prayer for my ultimate support. On September 25, 2007, I saw Dr. Bell to discuss my ever-worsening pain.

HISTORY OF PRESENT ILLNESS

[Sixty]-year-old woman with medical history significant for widespread CRPS [complex regional pain syndrome], RSD related bullous skin disorder, GERD, and odynophagia. Ema continues to follow regularly with Dr. Keith Bengston in PM&R [Physical Medicine and Rehabilitation] for her CRPS. She also follows periodically with Dr. Otley in Dermatology for RSD-related bullous skin disease.... She remains on the thalidomide, azathioprine, aloe vera, **holy anointing oil**, horse chestnut extract, and **prayer**.

Mrs. McKinley has a lengthy history of CRPS, going back at least 14 years. For much of that time, she has been followed regularly by Dr. Keith Bengston, who continues to manage and prescribe her pain medications. For the last several years, she has been on thalidomide and gradually escalating doses of MS Contin (extended relief morphine sulfate).

I have reviewed Dr. Bengston's clinical documents from his recent visits with Mrs. McKinley. It is apparent, as endorsed by the patient today, that she is becoming more desperate regarding her pain management issues. Numerous approaches to this have been provided and discussed by Dr. Bengston, **but unfortunately at this point we appear to be running out of options for her ...**

IMPRESSION/REPORT/PLAN

We discussed initiating a small dose of a tricyclic antidepressant such as nortriptyline ... This is helpful in the early stages for some RSD patients, **unfortunately we are at an advanced stage at this point**, but she is wishing to undertake a trial of this, after we discussed the typical side effects today.

We await her appointment at Pain Clinic for further recommendations regarding pain management options. Dr. Bengston is kindly facilitating this.

A couple months later, on November 12, 2007, they sent me to the pain management clinic for another assessment. After Dr. Richard

Rho reviewed my detailed and complex medical history, including my horrible reactions to medications, it became clear that even the experts in pain management couldn't help me.

HISTORY OF PRESENT ILLNESS

Briefly, Ms. McKinley is a 61-year-old female who has significant pain diffusely involving the majority of her body. She carries a diagnosis of CRPS which has involved her right upper extremity as well as other parts of her body secondarily, including her teeth. She has been receiving care under Dr. Bengston for the majority of 14 years or greater, and she has been through numerous trials of pain medications. She has drug intolerances to many medications which are listed in her allergies.

PHYSICAL EXAMINATION

General: Physical exam reveals a patient who appears her stated age. She has a somewhat bizarre posture where she is placing all of her weight on her left lower extremity while seated in a wheelchair bending dramatically over to the left. Her left hand is somewhat fixed in a fist position. Cognitively, she is intact.

IMPRESSION/REPORT/PLAN

Ms. McKinley certainly represents a severe, refractory case of CRPS. Given the chronicity, refractory nature of her condition, combined with her intolerance to many medications, **I have limited optimism that we will be able to significantly decrease her pain.**

As time went on, I continued to meet with my primary-care physician to discuss my progress — or, should I say, lack of progress — in managing my pain. During a visit on August 11, 2008, Dr. Bell confirmed my worst fear. Because the RSD was so advanced, we had exhausted drug options, which just left them with teaching me how to cope and live with the pain.

PHYSICAL EXAMINATION

General: Alert, fully oriented nondistressed 61-year-old woman seated in her wheelchair, leaning markedly to her left, baseline posture.

IMPRESSION/REPORT/PLAN

She continues on her longstanding chronic doses of MS Contin and Thalidomide as provided by Dr. Bengston in the PM&R clinic. Since her Pain Clinic visit in November 2007, she has gone through a course of adjuvant pain medications including nortriptyline, topiramate, and most recently Keppra. Unfortunately, she had little or no improvement with these. May have had a little bit of improvement with the Keppra, but she developed significant side effects earlier this summer, including allergic conjunctivitis ...

... The other development that Ema reports is that she is seeking another RSD specialist, as she feels that she and Dr. Bengston have exhausted their relationship after many, many years. She has not yet heard back from Dr. Bengston regarding his efforts to get her a physician in Pain Clinic (in the interval he continues to authorize thalidomide and MS Contin refills.)

PLAN

Understandably things remain very frustrating for Ema, particularly since she continues to suffer from significant headache and dental pain since weaning off the Keppra. As I have discussed with Ema today, **at this advanced stage of her RSD, we do not have the success in helping with symptoms that we sometimes do in the earlier stages of the diagnosis.** She has been very gallant about trying a number of adjuvant medications over the past 6–8 months, and I share in her frustration. **As we exhaust our pharmacologic options, the pain psychology aspect of our treatment becomes increasingly paramount in importance** ...

It is extremely difficult for Ema to participate in significant diagnostic testing, and over the years she has become more and more reluctant to undergo such testing. Understandably she has somewhat of a pessimistic attitude toward the value of such testing in the context of her progressive RSD symptomatology. In light of all of this, we have deferred further evaluation for now.

On January 21, 2009, I went to Dr. Arora, my gastroenterologist, because I felt a lump in the back of my throat, and whenever I swallowed liquids I felt a burning sensation. He ordered an EGD, but because of my allergies, I requested it without sedation.

HISTORY OF PRESENT ILLNESS

Ms. McKinley is a 62-year-old lady who has had wide-spread reflex sympathetic dystrophy symptoms following an accident several years ago. She is having worsening heartburn. She is having burning each time any liquids go down and has a substernal chest burning feeling regularly after taking her nutrition drink. She was doing reasonably well with Prilosec twice a day before meals, but now things have become worse. She is taking several Tums a day, and this does ease her burning, but she has to take this regularly. Her weight is now stabilized. In fact, it has increased since I last saw her in 2005 since she has been on thalidomide. She does not take any solid foods and just take[s] high-nutrition drinks only. She had a feeling of globus with a lump feeling in her throat, but food does not actually get stuck. No history of NSAID use.

She has very frequent episodes of vomiting, depending on the volume she takes. If she take[s] more than 3 or 4 ounces at a time, she will have regurgitation and vomiting that can be effortless. She has had episodes of aspiration with pneumonias in the past.

PHYSICAL EXAMINATION

General: She looks well. Cheerful. She is wheelchair bound, sitting clearly leaning to the left, unable to move neck and unable to use left arm at all. Left arm totally flexed.

Skin: erythema throughout.

Extremities: Left hand is clawed and immovable.

IMPRESSION/REPORT/PLAN

#1 Heartburn and globus

This is a very unfortunate story of a 62-year-old lady with widespread reflex sympathetic dystrophy who is wheelchair bound, at a[n] angle of 35–40 degrees and cannot move at all. I suspect she does have reflux, and this is aggravated by her body position. She has had problems with aspiration in the past. She has had respiratory distress with sedation, and she does not want to have any sedation. I think this is reasonable. **She does not want general anesthesia, and we have discussed doing an endoscopy under total non-sedation** (even without using Benzocaine spray). She is able to undergo dental extractions and drilling without any sedation, so I think we will do endoscopy unsedated. She will need to be in her wheelchair when they do this, and we will do this on the complex list. We will try and use the baby scope.

As I leaned on God to manage my pain, Charlie Bird continued to deal with the insurance issues and the bills they didn't want to pay. They even began to question my pain medications — specifically, the thalidomide. On April 29, 2009, Charlie wrote a letter to the opposing lawyer, explaining my need for thalidomide.

> You asked at the settlement conference the reasons why the thalidomide is considered necessary treatment. My understanding is that this medication increases the efficiency of the morphine, thus reducing the need for that medication. **She is in constant, extreme pain and with the high doses of morphine being less effective over time, this medication helps keep the morphine from reaching even higher, potentially lethal levels.**

Next, the insurance people argued that my thalidomide should be discontinued because it was considered an experimental drug for pain control. They claimed I didn't have RSD and that my pain was a psychological condition, all in my head. So Charlie rounded up the troops to get their expert opinions on my situation and on using thalidomide for my pain. On May 18, 2009, Dr. Bell stated:

> I have provided primary medical care to Mrs. Ema McKinley since February 2004. Her medical history is significant for widespread complex regional pain syndrome (CRPS), also known as reflex sympathetic dystrophy (RSD) initially diagnosed in 1993. Complications have included severe persistent chronic pain and RSD-related bullous skin disease.
>
> She was originally prescribed thalidomide on or around May 2002, on the recommendation of her Mayo Clinic CRPS specialists. Since my involvement with her care, she has remained on a stable dose of 400 mg once daily. **She has continued to have significant chronic pain during the past five years, with a slowly progressive decline in functional status ...**

My psychologist addressed their suggestion that my pain might be due to a psychological condition rather than RSD. She explained that I was actively seeking treatments to improve my symptoms—not trying to stay sick like the opposing side said. She also explained how my faith helped me through all my medical challenges. On August 21, 2009, Dr. Cindy Smith, licensed psychologist, stated:

> Ema is concerned about her health and continues to consider all the medical interventions presented to her, even after some of the interventions resulted in the worsening of her symptoms and limitations. It is true that she is cautious when considering physical interventions because several past interventions resulted in the worsening of her pain and limitations ... One might be tempted to consider her positive attitude as a lack of concern or in some way secondary gain, but it is my clinical opinion that **her strong faith in God has allowed her to maintain such an attitude in the face of extreme pain and limits** ... Because of Ema's strong reliance upon her God, she has successfully managed chronic pain by following her doctor's orders with medications, maintaining appropriate activity level and resting to deal with physical factors. **She maintains emotional stability utilizing relaxation and meditating/praying, which brings her hope for the present and future.** Finally, her faith in God allows her to deal with the grieving of her progressive losses associated with RSD/CRPS and the challenges of her daily life. Her thoughts are focused on her God, His will for her life and what she can do for others. This focus allows distraction from her pain and losses to an adaptive attitude and feeling that she can control her focus to help others ...

On August 31, 2009, Dr. Bengston confirmed for the opposing side that I did, in fact, have RSD. He also pointed out that there weren't other treatment options for me. They had already tried everything—but had no success.

Apparently, there has [sic] still been questions as to the patient's underlying diagnosis. Clearly, the patient has fulfilled the Minnesota Worker's Compensation criteria for reflex sympathetic dystrophy (better known as complex regional pain syndrome) ... In addition, by current medical standards, the patient clearly has met the criteria for complex regional pain syndrome as established by the International Association for the Study of Pain.

I have read the recommendations ... of [the doctor who did an independent medical examination] ... I do agree with his opinions about what is the proper treatment for someone in Ms. McKinley's condition. Unfortunately, those treatments have already been tried in the past and failed ... she has already been through these in the earlier stages of her disease and unfortunately continued to progress despite attempts at this multidisciplinary approach ...

The patient has a significant truncal contracture that has developed over the years with a scoliotic curve of the thoracolumbar spine. The assumption has always been that this is a manifestation of the CRPS and in general related to the asymmetric involvement of the trunk muscles. **Certainly, no other etiology has ever been found in regard to her postural changes and I suspect that, given the chronicity of these changes, they are irreversible.**

On September 14, 2009, Charlie Bird put together a thorough and detailed summary of my medical and legal history for the judge who would be evaluating my case. Here's how he described my situation in the letter:

If anything is established in this case beyond dispute, it is that the employee suffers from one of the worst cases of RSD and consequential injuries that have ever been brought. She is crippled in multiple extremities, multiple organs and multiple systems ... She suffers from intractable, chronic extreme pain. There is no alternative treatment. She can only hope for relief from pain and no cure is available. To that end, the doctors are offering compassion and pain relief. Doctors are prescribing what can only be described as "end-of-life" dosages of morphine for pain control. This is a drug that results in rising levels of tolerance and there is a risk that prescribing ever-increasing doses could cause significant deleterious side-effects ...

The employee's condition has continued to deteriorate over the years. The use of pain control medication is not curative, but is instead palliative. The body parts that are involved in the work-related injury continue to expand and it is reasonably expected that her symptoms, overall, will generally progress downward over time ...

Despite the best efforts of my lawyer and doctors, the insurance arguments successfully blocked my ongoing use of thalidomide. So, during the fall of 2010, my doctors weaned me off it and increased my morphine. Sadly, the doctors were out of options. And as Charlie Bird stated in his letter to the judge, they gave up trying to cure me a long time ago. On April 1, 2011, in my final visit with Dr. Bell before the miracle, we mostly talked about medication and the fact that there was nothing else to try.

PHYSICAL EXAMINATION

Alert, fully oriented, 64-year-old woman seated in her wheelchair in her typical posture leaning far laterally towards the left.

IMPRESSION/REPORT/PLAN

She was on a stable dose of MS Contin [morphine] and thalidomide for many years but was tapered off the thalidomide completely during the fall of 2010. We continued her at that time on high doses of MS Contin, and we attempted to modify her regimen with fentanyl patch, which did not improve her pain management and was noted to cause unpleasant side effect.

So for the last several months she has been on a stable dose of MS Contin of 1600 mg daily in divided doses. This alone, since the discontinuation of the thalidomide, does not provide adequate pain management to the level that she was receiving previously.

We had a lengthy discussion regarding ongoing narcotic pain management. **At this point we have nothing additional to offer her** but could try an increased dose of her MS Contin. She has always used this in a responsible fashion.

We will trial a higher dose, and I have rewritten her prescription for MS Contin 100 mg tablets to take 10 twice daily.

After this visit, my morphine dosage went up to a whopping 2000 mg daily. The doctors didn't know what else to do for me. Dr. Bell continued to renew my prescriptions, but other than a couple visits to the eye doctor and dermatologist, the next few months were quiet on both the medical and legal fronts. That is, until my Christmas Eve miracle.

In the weeks and months following my miracle, I returned to many of my doctors so they could hear my remarkable story and reevaluate my dramatically changed body and physical condition. I set up my first appointment with Dr. Bell, my primary-care doctor since 2004, and I got in to see him on January 4, 2012, eleven days after my miraculous healing.

HISTORY OF PRESENT ILLNESS

Patient's pain was reported using the Numeric pain scale. Patient/caregiver rates pain at a 6–7. Ms. McKinley comes with her caregivers to discuss medication and related concerns in the context of her longstanding, widespread, complex regional pain syndrome. Her last visit with me was April 1, 2011. Her medical history is significant for widespread CRPS, RSD-related bullous skin disorder, GERD, odynophagia, and probable right upper extremity carpal tunnel syndrome. In the past she has also followed with Dr. Bengston, in PM&R; and Dr. Otley, in Dermatology. Also seen by Dr. Rho, in Pain Clinic, on November 12, 2007. She continues on chronic high-dose narcotics for pain management. Her thalidomide was tapered and discontinued late 2010. She comes in today to review medications and related concerns as detailed below in the IRP.

PHYSICAL EXAMINATION

General: **Alert, fully oriented, nondistressed 65-year-old woman who was standing upright when I entered the room**. She was easily fatigued in this position but able to walk a few steps with standby assistance to her wheelchair. Has an upright posture in her wheelchair.

IMPRESSION/REPORT/PLAN

Astonishingly, she was standing independently as I entered the room today. Her previous chronic posture has been wheelchair bound, leaning far laterally toward the left. She had been in that wheelchair-bound posture since my initial meeting with her in 2004, gradually worsening. She relates an extraordinary story of how she regained her ability to stand this past Christmas Eve. She accidentally fell out of her wheelchair that day while alone at home and spent several hours on the floor in agony and crying out. Her story of how she was able to regain her feet and stand up that evening is amazing. She is accompanied during today's visit by her longtime attendant, Cathy, and her son, Jason, of Rochester. They see her on a daily basis and were equally astounded by her recovery.

She fatigues easily, and we have discussed arranging some physical therapy for her for improvement of lower extremity strength, endurance, balance, and gait training. She is interested in water aerobics and eventually in horseback riding as in the remote past, before her illness, she assisted children with these activities.

She also has concerns about her diet. For many years her primary intake has been nutritional drinks as she has not been able to hold other types of food down. I am confident that eventually we can get her on more solid foods, but she is reluctant to try yet, preferring to proceed with physical therapy in the immediate future.

She still has significant pain which we are managing with high-dose narcotics chronically. She is adherent to her current plan of care, and we will make no adjustment in her narcotic plan at this time. Eventually we should be able to taper this down hopefully.

Plan for her now is to arrange the physical therapy, continue current medicines, continue current nutritional drinks, with her plan to contact me as she becomes more willing and ready to advance her diet. We are all amazed with her recent improvement.

Two weeks later, on January 18, 2012, I saw Dr. Kathryn Stolp, the head of physical therapy, to develop a plan to rehabilitate my muscles. Dr. Stolp also gave me a complete physical examination to evaluate my spine, joints, gait, motor skills, and mental status. This provided a comprehensive picture of my transformed body and life — just a few weeks after my miracle.

HISTORY OF PRESENT ILLNESS

Right-handed woman who had an accident and was hung upside down at work from her left foot and ankle for 2.5 hours unconscious. This then led to a more global pain problem involving her entire body including her eyes, teeth, and jaw. She has carried the diagnosis of chronic regional pain syndrome for many years. Today she brings photos of how she was in terms of sitting in her wheelchair where she lived for the past 20+ [sic] years. She sat in her wheelchair full time and in fact slept in her wheelchair and she sat flexed at the waist in a very distorted posture with her left hand closed shut and she was only able to use her right upper limb. She would slide from the chair onto a toilet with grab bars and bathed via sponge baths because water from a shower spray was excruciatingly painful. She was stable in this condition all of this time despite multiple therapeutic efforts. She was totally dependent in self care and was not able to swallow solids so has lived on high calorie nutrition drinks but has not had to have a PEG [feeding tube into stomach].

On Christmas Eve morning at 1:00 AM, she went to turn in her chair and her wheel became trapped. She fell out of the chair. She laid on the floor for 8 hours and screamed at the top of her lungs the whole time and was not able to call anyone and prayed to God. She felt God enter her body and straightened her hand and foot out, and new flesh appeared where she had macerated skin. This phenomenon then spread to her spine and she was able to flip over and lie straight in a supine position. Moments later, she saw a beautiful white robe that was very bright but without a face that her human eyes could barely see. Then God knelt beside her, asked for her hand, and he took both hands and stood her up on both feet. She reports that her bones were cracking all over and she started walking down the hallway and she was very ataxic and incoordinated [sic].

Since then, she has found that her chronic severe headache is about 50% less. The total body burning is still present in the left hand and right hand and both feet. She has some bilateral hip and back pain remaining. She is walking short distances. She needs assistance getting up. She has some joint tightness that seems to limit her. She feels her balance is poor and needs to hold the walls or furniture. She still feels the "RSD is still part of me in terms of the burning pain" but is hopeful that therapy can now help her. She also feels that she has an echo in her ears since sitting upright. She still drops things.

SOCIAL HISTORY

Live[s] alone. Family members and a PCA provide about 70 hours a week of care which has continued since the miracle because of the hand weakness and imbalance.

PHYSICAL EXAMINATION

General: Well-developed, well-nourished individual in no acute distress.

Spine: She actually has **quite good cervical and lumbar range of motion**. She is generally painful to touch and touching tends to result in persistent tingling in most areas.

Joints: Seated, I was unable to elevated [sic] her arms past 90 degrees of abduction. When supine, I was able to achieve full abduction of the right shoulder which was painful at end range and when testing the left supine, I believe she was more guarded and I was not able to elevated [sic] past 90 degrees. She clearly has heel cord contractures and probably hip and knee flexion contractures as well. **Elbows, wrists, fingers move well.**

Gait: Wearing two inch heels. Requires **assistance to stand from chair and then walks with a fairly stiff, broad-based**

gait with more stiffness left than right leg and limited arm swing. Turns well. When returning to sit, even sitting back onto elevated plinth, she flops down with some assistance onto the plinth.

Mental: Alert, appropriate, excellent historian.

Motor: Normal right upper and lower limb strength. − 1 throughout left side with some give away but I believe there may be some weakness there which I did not mention to her.

Sensation: Joint position sense is intact. I am not completely certain about pin sensation which seemed patchy and non-dermatomal. Some hyperalgesia but not much allodynia.

Deep tendon reflexes: May be more slightly brisk on left than right. Babinski nonreactive.

IMPRESSION/REPORT/PLAN

This is an extraordinary case. Fortunately, she is now much more mobile than she has been for years. Regardless her exact diagnosis, she is undoubtedly profoundly deconditioned and does have joint contractures and in fact, **it is amazing the joints move as well as they do.** I will have her seen by physical and occupational therapy in our functional gait/behavioral shaping program ... I suspect she will have to progress through therapy very slowly and cautiously perhaps even starting with something very simple such as passive or active assistive range and stretching with some beginning core strengthening and then building from there ...

On March 30, 2012, I saw Dr. Otley, the dermatologist who had treated me for more than ten years, including when the RSD sores erupted on my legs and they wanted to amputate my right leg. I wanted him to see me standing upright and mobile, and then fully examine me.

HISTORY OF PRESENT ILLNESS

A 65-year-old woman with a long and complicated history of chronic regional pain syndrome complicated by cellulitis; DVT; milia; molluscum; dermatitis; intertrigo; and a bullous disorder of an undefined nature, probably bullous CRPS. **She has been contracted in a wheelchair for as long as I have known her with severe immobility. She has been bent over at the waist with poor functioning of her hands and feet** ... I first evaluated her in 2000 when she had recurrent ulcerations and nodules ... We primarily provided supportive care along with some anti-inflammatories ...

She relays a history on New Year's Eve [sic] of 2011 of falling from her wheelchair and spending eight agonizing hours on the floor in pain. This was followed by the appearance of what she feels was God. She saw a bright robe with human hands but no face. She interacted with this apparition operation, and her joints were straightened, her skin was loosened, her hand was released from contractures and her spine was straightened, and she walked with this vision. Since that time, she has been very weak but has resumed walking and is upright and able to sleep in a lying straight position. Her life has been transformed, and she feels it is a miracle.

PHYSICAL EXAMINATION

Skin: An upright, straight-spined, noncontracted individual who is able to walk with no assistance but with hesitation. She is alert and oriented and conversant as usual. Her skin feels very normal on her hands, and she has mobility of her hand joints. She is able to move her legs normally ... overall, things look amazingly well.

IMPRESSION/REPORT/PLAN

Her skin had been doing better more recently but certainly, **it is amazing that she has had a dramatic recovery from her chronic contractures and immobility due to her complex regional pain syndrome.** Her description of her miraculous recovery with an apparition is remarkable. At this point, her skin does not need anything other than moisturizers and occasional anti-inflammatory creams if she gets a recurrence of her hives or irritant dermatitis … All questions were answered, and I voiced sincere pleasure with the dramatic recovery of her health.

Timeline

October 23, 1946	Ema McKinley born in Waterloo, Iowa.
April 10, 1993	Accident at Garretts department store.
April 12, 1993	Ema wakes up in St. Mary's Hospital, Rochester, Minnesota.
May 20, 1993	Ema diagnosed with Reflex Sympathetic Dystrophy (RSD).
July–August 1993	Ema participates in physical therapy.
September 1993	Ema returns to work at Garretts, part time.
January 1995	Ema collapses walking to work, never returns to Garretts.
January 26, 1995	Ema signs retainer agreement with attorney Charlie Bird.
July 1995	Ema attends a pain management clinic.
November 1995	Ema's chiropractor can no longer help her as RSD advances.
November 1995	Ema's left hand begins to claw.
December 24, 1995	Ema's last full meal with solid foods.
February 1996	Ema is confined to a wheelchair.
January 6, 1997	Workers' Compensation Court ruling in favor of Ema.

January 1998	Court settlement reached with insurance.
September 26, 1998	Ema moves into her new townhome.
July 1999	Head attachment added to Ema's wheelchair.
September 30– October 3, 1999	Twin Cities for second opinion, rushed to ER, mild heart attack.
October 4–6, 1999	Ema's brief battle with depression.
December 2000– December 2001	Connor chosen as child ambassador for March of Dimes.
Fall 2003	Ema has respiratory failure, rushed to ER, near-death experience.
Spring 2004	RSD sores appear on Ema's legs.
September 18, 2004	Ema participates in Minnesota Dermatological Society meeting.
September 2004	Dr. Otley recommends amputation of Ema's right leg.
December 2004	Ema's RSD sores, infection, and blood clots clear up on right leg.
August 11, 2005	Dr. Tamara Vos-Draper recommends modifying wheelchair due to excessive overhang.
September 25, 2007	Dr. Bell: "We appear to be running out of options for her."
January 23, 2009	Ema undergoes endoscopy of upper digestive tract without sedation.
October 7, 2009	Dr. Bengston: "We might not find anything that is actually fixable."

October–December 2010	Ema has extreme difficulty adjusting to 1600 mg morphine.
April 1, 2011	Dr. Bell increases Ema's morphine to 2000 mg.
December 24, 2011	9:00 a.m.: Christmas Eve miracle, Jesus heals Ema.
December 24, 2011	8:00 p.m.: Ema surprises sons and grand-sons on Christmas Eve.
December 25, 2011	Ema surprises Cathy, Daddy, and other family members.
January 4, 2012	Ema surprises Dr. Bell, is upright, walking, using her hand. Healed.
January 18, 2012	Ema sees Dr. Stolp for exam and restarts physical therapy.
May 16–17, 2012	Ema's story featured on KAAL-TV, ABC News, Rochester, Minnesota.
October 2012– February 2013	Ema reduces daily morphine from 1600 mg to 0 mg.
December 25, 2012	Ema's story featured on *700 Club*, Virginia Beach, Virginia.
February 15, 2013	Ema speaks at Madonna Towers, Rochester, Minnesota.
June 28, 2013	Ema speaks at Salvation Army Rehabilita-tion Center, Minneapolis, Minnesota.